I0758000

CHAMPION GUIDES

Fifth Edition of Psych Classic with Images

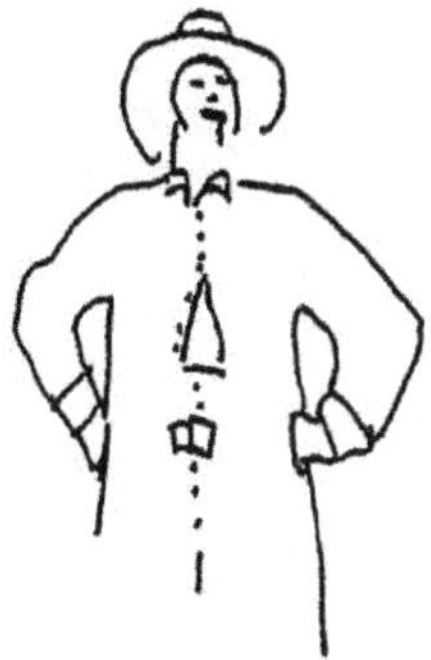

Written and Illustrated By
Karen Kellock Ph.D

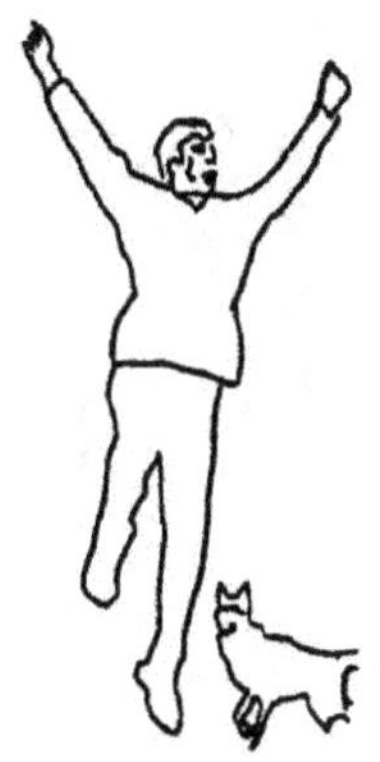

*I dedicate this book series to
children and animals:
the innocent will of God, and to all
God's Elect. To make an amazing new dent:
fast (fly), separate and repent!*

FORMULA:

All success attraction
All disease obstruction
All recovery elimination

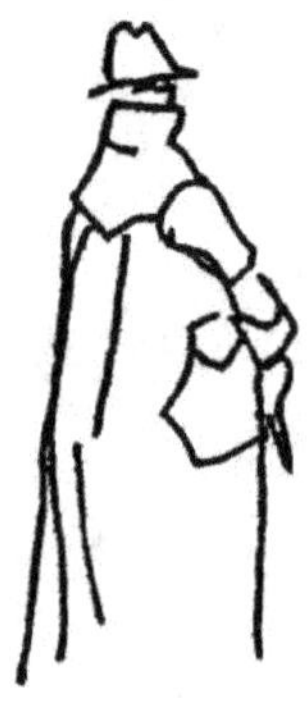

You must fast on all three

OBSTRUCTIONS:

People
Habit
Food

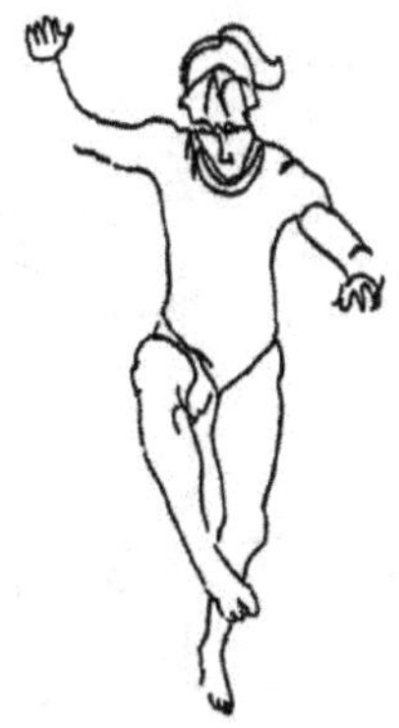

The DAILY FAST

is always rewarded

Champion Guides Series

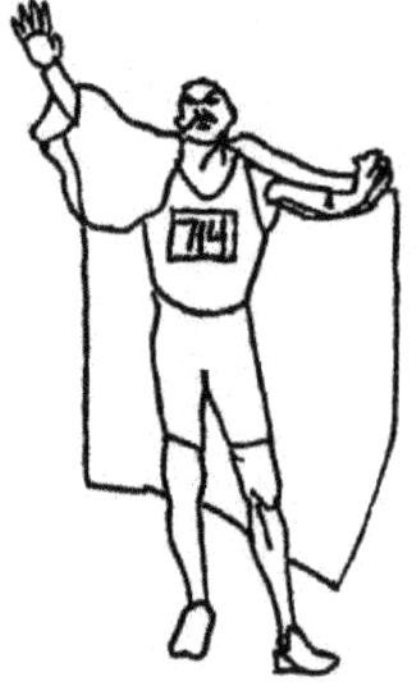

Manual for Superior Men

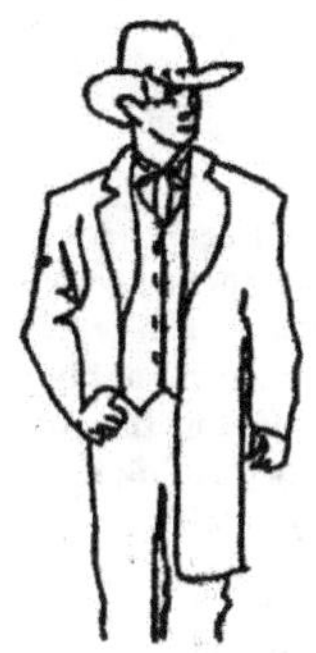

Welcome to the highest life possible:

DAILY FASTARIANISM

**It is a magic door you step into by the mere decision to fast on people, habit and food.
The superior man knows that whatever the problem, just by fasting he enters this door
where his foes fall to the floor, he changes to the core and to the fast he says "I want more"**

Sun-moon-stars. Few are clear enough to enjoy the pleasures of the higher senses (who but the superior man could, since the world is fogged with distraction?) But there is a way: fasting creates a psychic opening and then mass attractions to the true self. As part of nature the Creative Act evolves through cycles which cannot be rushed. But for those with the courage to work and patience to wait the entire act together with the reward itself will fall together in a fabric. It is the FAST which provides this link to success. Who but the superior man could wait patiently until everything comes to him?

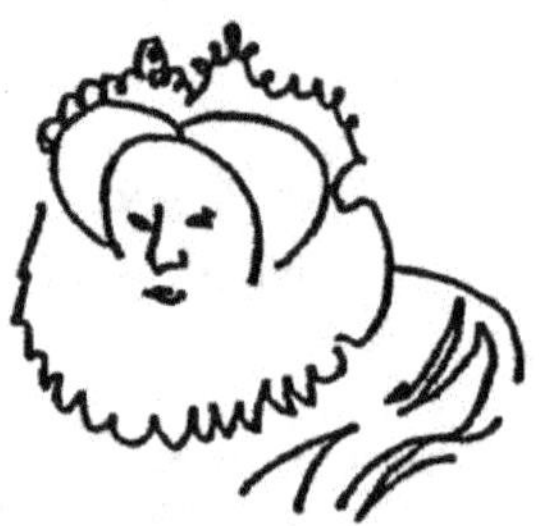

Karen Kellock: Recovery through
Solitude And Daily Fasting on People, Habit and Food

CHAMPION GUIDES

PART ONE:
PEOPLE AND HABITS

CHAMPION GUIDES

PART ONE

Purified Genius Comes Out, Having Dissolved All
Sick Systems and Sin Cycles

In the Act of Creation Koestler showed how landmark discoveries link with history—as part of nature, would this not be true? We all have a unique talent, the seed of a creative act inside--but it's a mere potential. It must be developed to blossom into world-changing power. This natural process in man is blocked by obstruction: people, habits and food. But if pure, the creative act evolves through cycles: it sprouts, moves into place and completes itself naturally. Timing is all: the minute the act is complete the link appears. Just by fasting and doing what comes naturally our true genius comes through: we do magical work for magical pay. The test of discovery is: does it work?

PART TWO

Paleo science, not vegan dogma: Human functioning has more to
do with released obstruction than vitaminerals.

Fruit-Fat-Fastarianism

Karen Kellock DAILY FASTING as it relates to psychology and winning. How worldly and satisfying, the fruit and fat daily fasting or fruit-fat-fastarianism. As an ex-vegan fruitarian she found total recovery through this "Heavenly Triangle". This is paleo science not vegan dogma which for me brought failure to thrive and dissolved teeth. Like the cats, man needs animal fats (fauna). But it's the Daily Fast which is always rewarded so fast each day. You'll see your digestion, assimilation, elimination (and thus appearance) improve as all hunger dissolves. All your problems you'll find this solves. There will be complete recovery through solitude and Daily Fasting on People, Habit and Food.

Karen Kellock Ph.D.

BLUE GENIUS

*It's a World Obstruction: Being Ignored
Hated and Misunderstood*

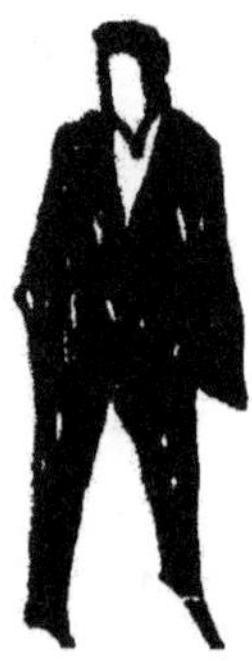

We all have unique gifts which would make us champions in our field were it not for the obstructions in our lives. How to be a champion: release your obstruction then attain the spiritual skies as you rise up in your field. We're all potential geniuses but it's only a dormant potential. It must be developed to blossom to world success. This theory of how to rise up has one very simple formula: all disease is obstruction, all recovery is elimination and all success is attraction. There are three obstructions: people, habit and food. Release your obstruction and you will snap to your goals waiting in the wings.

It is natural for genius to unfold but in the world it meets resistances. Blocked genius is blue: before it comes to its own it remains an as-yet-unrecognized, would-be or "wanna-be" and that just isn't good enough. To be a world success you must hit the bull's eye. The way you get to the promised land is to release these obstructions in your life:

(1) People. Be very careful with whom you associate lest they contaminate your aura and pull you down. Many "symptoms" are just appropriate reactions to sick systems which maintain that problem. True success entails a period of separation and then reconnection. (2) Habit. You must eradicate--give up, turn from, repent of--all bad habits. You know which ones I mean because underneath we always know better. Due to the laws of energy these habits will automatically degrade from your best as they recycle energy in outworn channels. Through habit we're stuck in ruts that literally blind us from the light illuminating the path to success. (3) Food. Most people are physically filled with superfluity—debris-

seen-as-fat--having a diet of unnatural modern foods which are biologically unusable and thus stored in the fat "false body." Genius succeeds through the "higher paleo" Neolithic diet of fruit, fats and the daily fast. All other foods are evolutionarily discordant: grains, beans, other starches and sugar. Man has been a fruit and fat-eater from the beginning. Fruit is a purifier, fat is a re-builder and the fat and fiber (in nuts, avocados or fauna) are colon-happy eliminators.

PEOPLE

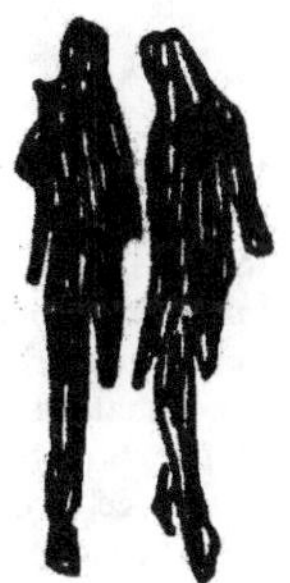

It is frightening how much people are like animals in their group behavior. People can be cruel as they hold you down. Being part of a sick system degrades as manipulation and control destroys life and destiny. The would-be genius must manage associations and insulate from all ungodly control. He must cut his life into his own pattern and let no one dissuade him from it. Having eliminated all distractions he can then focus and achieve his goal--the unleashing of all his true genius talents which are totally unique or they aren't true genius.

Only the True Self which transcends culture, age and gender must prevail--this is the perfect blueprint for success. We must first detach from old or evil props then develop from the inside-out. Detaching from sick society we can then embark on an exciting inner journey to the True Self as God designed. Do not be adapted to the present age--its superficial customs and modes of thought--but be transformed by the renewal of your mind. Then you will prove the will of God which is your genius.

True enlightenment is not "going with the flow" or adapting but insulating from the human herd and then unfolding in your own stream. Here there is no competition just the burgeoning of raw talent into success. Insulation is the mark of the superior man--he creates his own universe and adapts to no one. He makes his environment reflect his personality so his personality will be enhanced.

HABIT

Einstein proved it's all just energy. If clear and open to this source our lives are filled with creative action and opulent abundance. We are remunerated for our talents and unique genius. But bad habits block this process as they recycle energy into ruts long dead. Sin blocks. Having turned from these useless ruts--which make us poor, ugly and mean--the duality in man becomes unified into one-pointed mind power so now we hit the mark automatically. When stuck in ruts and cycles we block the light revealing completion. With final repentance the historical saints instantly shot up to world greatness after many fruitless and frustrating silent years.

FOOD

In the last twenty years our culture has fallen into a pit of obesity bringing despair and confusion. This is not so much gluttony but the wrong diet. Only by eating the fruit and fat are we hitting the right groove, as these foods are so potent only mouse-meals are required enabling long periods of fasting or frugal eating each day. The pure fruitarian diet requires much eating (high-water and calorie-sparse) and brings on cravings, and the farmer diet of flour pasty foods and sugars raise insulin so that we "wear" everything we eat. This starchy diet has been our reaction to the fear of dietary fat--fat phobia---as we have substituted animal fat with so much starch like pasta, rice, bread cereals and tubers. The paleo diet using animal fat (fauna) and fruits makes us strong and handsome blueprints of God.

FASTING

All through history the sages and saints used fasting as a method to overcome enemies and achieve success. It has always been the way to get to God's power. In part two you will see very simple ways of fasting daily, like just skipping dinner. You will be amazed at the exhilaration and the revelation that comes with just one meal skipped. Fast and you're using the oldest and most efficient method used by man to perform miracles and complete old cycles while beginning new ones.

1

GENIUS IS HELD DOWN

by People, Habits and Food.
Repent for Success and Bliss

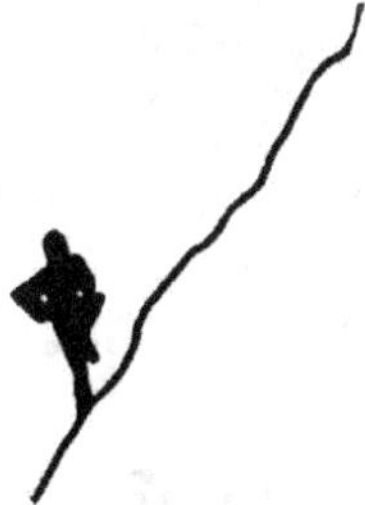

Genius is held down by obstruction: people, habit and food. Because of his differences the would-be genius can be stigmatized and held down by groups firstly and then by his own addictions to avoid anxiety from persecution, and if he eats wrong he is then held down by his own inner debris. This is a very simple theory. Just know the three obstructions and remove them, knowing the glory that lies ahead. You will then snap to all your unrealized goals waiting in the wings.

When obstructed there is a heaviness to the personality. People are cluttered with the nonessential and useless distractions. To succeed, eliminate the non-essential in body, mind and group. Leave all this heaviness behind--press on to what lies ahead! Rid of people problems you become a sage or monk finally able to accomplish something. Rid of bad habits you become a prosperous saint, and rid of inner debris--the superfluous flesh from wrong eating--you're a savant with a miraculous body well into old age. Living this way--truly free--will make you ecstatically happy and productive the rest of your long life. As you leave the outer behind and implode into the inner you'll become far more productive and useful the older you get. In your eighties you will just begin to maximize your mental powers for as the physical wanes the mystical and mental will increase to the same degree-so look forward with glee. All the morbid cultural fears about age are the opposite to the truth. Never forget this expression: OP-TRUTH for all popular notions are false!

PROCRUSTEAN CONFORMITY

We are all taught to conform to the same mold: the standard one in society. Procrusteas was a giant who stretched or amputated his captives to fit his iron bed: procrustean conformity. Having to adapt this way splits us from our true selves, where the joy lies. Losing the self is a homesick existence that paradoxically makes us seek out others more, thus losing self more. The bull's-eye to success is going solo. To go solo is to be with God-- separate is sanctified, holy. To tow the line to conform to other people is a life of missed opportunity and lost miracles. These are happening every second but you can never know them lost in loony logorrhea: word salad or silly conversations where the trivial is indistinguishable from the important. That's society. Just listen for awhile and you will hear it.

Do you love people? Then help them to transcend the obstacles to creativity in dense herds and become their True Self. Then they're a shining light and exemplar to the race. To conform and make others do likewise just maintains the mundane social world--the bland, boring, banal, benign. Having transcended the resistances which I will describe you become cosmic: influenced by God's creative spirit, not by other people. People will only hold you down.

MAN THE ADAPTIVE ANIMAL

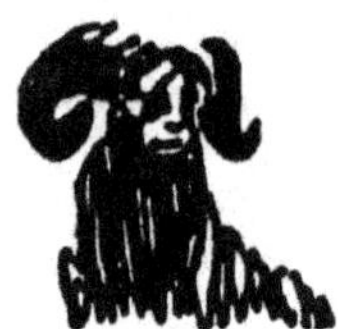

Man is an adaptive animal--he adapts to his environment. When it is sick he mal-adapts by becoming sick. These mal-adaptations are his obstructions to health and wealth in a life of frenetic stressful laboring. In contrast, cosmic man does nothing. He attracts what he is. Because he has peace he has total power. Having emptied himself of all obstructions he has become an irresistible magnet to all good attractions while automatically repelling all-bad. Spiritually right his work becomes effortless as it flows through with "holy spirit ease." Rid of obstructions he rules by attraction. This paradigm shift to ENERGY has one general formula for all life sciences:

Obstructions make us miserable, angry and depressed:

CHAMPION GUIDES

PEOPLE (sick systems)
HABIT (sin cycles)
FOOD (superfluity)

All success attraction
All disease obstruction
All recovery elimination

Before conversion life is chaotic and dark--made DENSE from one or all of these obstructions:

PEOPLE

It is frightening how much people are like animals in their group behavior. They can really hold you down as maintaining the system--the status quo---becomes the glue of groups. Systems maintain themselves through mental conformity. People gain identity in relation to others so they must "keep each other in their place" to keep identity intact. Since identity is relational people will destroy others to maintain it. This is why sick family systems will keep the "patient" down and sabotage recovery--for the sake of their own identity.

HABIT

Bad habits maintain bad memories. Bad memories in turn become the cue triggering the craving to sin. Giving into the same old habit simply reinforces the memory--which continues to degrade. To mature to genius and success one must transcend the past completely and then keep the slate clean each day, lest memory compel the repetition of old cycles. Any temptation habitually denied will cease to exist, but will gain stronger hold each time we give in.

FOOD

Most food creates debris: dead matter with weight coming from the wrong diet of all but the natural (Neolithic) foods from the beginning: fruit and fat. The vegetables are also paleo but man is not folivorous (leaf- or plant-eating) so these are really for other animals. Meat-eating is also paleo but "higher paleo" is for those who wish a harmless raw diet of fruit and fat (like avocados, nuts or cheese). Man is a fat-frugivore: the fruit cleans, the fat rebuilds. Man is like a cat—he needs fat for the brain, heart, glands and skin. In the modern diet all this is reversed as the animal fat is replaced by starch foods which are biologically unusable and stored in fatty water pockets and other superfluous debris. What unsightly flesh we humans display when in favor or rice or beans we avoid the cheese-tray!

Constantly elevated insulin from starch and sugar (carb) leaves the body full of disease-storage and a suppressed immune system. Protein deficiency degrades immunity even more. All of the degenerative diseases of civilization—hypertension, coronary heart disease, diabetes, obesity and atherosclerosis are due to the high-carb diet which puts the body in fat storage mode and constricts the arteries. Eating modern food means we wear everything we eat. Nuts are as dry but they are paleo so the body knows how to use them. Nothing is more delicious than the triadic diet of fruits and their Red Salads, nuts, cheese and olive oil. You'll need one meal or two meals six hours apart—have a happy breakfast of raisins and nuts and a lunch with Red Salad (tomatoes, red bells, lemon/olive oil dressing) with your avocado or fauna: cheese, fish or egg condiments. Then fast for your dinner for human growth hormone is elevated with fasting at night—and thus the body does a total repair, a youthification into beauty. Do you dare enjoy life this much for the rest of your days on this beautiful earth?

FAT-PHOBIA GOES AGAINST YA

Carb-addiction is the malady of the masses. The carb-addict loves starches and sugar, thinks about food constantly and can't stop eating. He is always hungry and often irritable--they go together as insulin creates psych-pathology. The elevated insulin forces the body to retain water and salt, closes in all the airways and arteries and leads to hypertension, moodiness violence and brain fog. The sugar and starch brings sleepiness and depression while fat is a brain-stimulant. After one goes straight (and streamlined) with a high protein and fat diet along with fruit his body is relieved of all this superfluity, the water drains out and he feels energetic, happy, even. These gut-dense potent foods like nuts or cheese enables daily fasting for 18 hours and this is a most creative lifestyle in which one is easily able to fast all day due to potent foods which require so little to sustain while keeping the gut flat. Then the superior man takes fruitarian vacations to quick-cleanse the system, often combined with short fasts like "worthy week-enders" in which he is most happy—more so each time he embarks on the faster's inner journey.

THEY ALL GO TOGETHER

All three obstructions reinforce each other. The "bad tone" from constipation or insulin elevation is an uncomfortable condition which brings heaviness to the personality, loss of energy, fascination and stability. It is pure obstruction as fat is continuously laid on. Starch and sugar turns genius to jello. The results are people problems and other bad habits to self-medicate the constant dull drag. From flabby to firm—changing your diet also changes your habits and associates. When this continuous insulin elevation and constipation is eliminated the result is clarity. With clear nerves and synapses we gain the ecstatic birthright of humans. With skill and new co-ordination from fat-moistened brain, heart, glands and tissues we become the true genius we were created to be.

GENIUS GOES UP OR WAY DOWN

The genius is in conflict with the petty negative forces trying to pull him down to something *they* can understand. His job is to develop the moral strength to overcome these resistances, rise up in spite of them and make an amazing new dent in the world. This tremendous feat can only be accomplished through moral purity. Impurity will weaken and a sudden rise to success will be   followed by an overnight fall. Sin creates arrogance and arrogance always precedes downfall!

The Bible is clear on the evil of these latter days: men would be lovers of self, lovers of money, arrogant, malicious, gossipers, without self-control, brutal and vicious haters of good, treacherous, reckless, conceited, steeped in forms of religion but still unholy, captivators of weak women and always learning but never coming to the truth. In this sour state of mind people scapegoat those different from them. What this means is that in all cultures genius in his primitive state has much to overcome, simply because his radical differences prevent adaptation to dense conformity. In this generation high-tech progress camouflages the severe degeneration in other areas: mind, spirit, body, family, and knit of society. Genius is a rose hitting a hard brick wall so most give up or die through self-destructive addictions to avoid anxiety. Through this book and site you will rise up to a position of new-found power—just through knowledge of what is going on in the human herd which maintains cohesion by destroying differences.

GENIUS MUST BE CHAMPION

Genius must learn to be a champion standing out in a sea of sharks. He must be a brilliant radiant life reflecting the Creator's blueprint--his True Self, not led by puny finite darkened minds of men but inspired by the inerrant Godly force transcending all culture and silly human fashions--of thoughts, morality, customs. Genius must learn self-gentleness and to deal with these times by becoming sensitive to the works of God—nature, seasons, love, beauty and genius in himself and others. Becoming Godly brings awareness of the futility of the lives of the ungodly--no progress, failing, vanity, carnality and misery.

ENTER EINSTEIN

This theory uses Einstein Energy Theories as the basis of the matrix. The major energy formula is from his Field Theory:

1. It is all just energy.
2. All gravity is attraction.
3. There is no time or space

Einstein has proven that everything in the universe is just energy at different rates of speed. This is creative energy. If man is open to this energy source he sings, he dances, he soars. His creative genius--a dormant seed in all men--awakens to make an amazing new dent in the world. As open and clear he now attracts all and becomes a success against overwhelming odds. The mature genius has bliss--freedom from obstruction. He has learned how people can hold him down, how bad habits degrade through dead repetition blocking the creative and how physical obstruction through wrong eating obstructs the creative ecstasy leading to perfect work. The three obstructions are simple to know--the budding genius reader is asked to answer the test of all science discovery: Does it Work?

ADAPTATION TO THE SOCIAL WORLD

This book is to the herd, about the herd, for the herd. We are all being held down by it. We are it! The herd is not a person but a mentality which equates being different as being bad. The Bible reads in Psalms: Fear every voice which calls you to partake of the world. You are _in_ the world but not _of_ it. Keep this distinction clear. Neurosis and addiction are ways of coping with the mixed signals of sick systems and society. These are hostile environments characterized by contradictions--the only way of "fitting " is by "slipping." People's misjudgments of others may become a program or script of the other's behavior--he becomes what they say he is.

This is nothing new--it's been around since time began and all societies/families are involved. To those denying this sad social fact the notion may bring fear. Good--for it is the shock of recognition of cultural/family patterns keeping you down, depressed and drunk which will bring your psychic opening into clarity: the Greatness of your True Self. Through the following pages you will see that you are not to blame for all mad or bad behavior is a mal-adaptation to a sick system--a hostile environment. With this knowledge you must now get free to do your work. Together we can work things out.

Clear, you will multi-adapt to an ever-changing universe, not mal-adapt through disease, blindness and being "hooked". The True Self is spirit, which is energy--it cannot be held down without severe and painful results. Releasing blocked energy brings self-expression-- the raw talents in the fine design--and perfect success. Genius is held down by prideful puffed-up powers exalting themselves above God. Thinking they are God (new age slogan) they are jealous of the talents (God's energy) coming through you.   It is a spiritual war between clear and dense (good and evil). The involvement of human networks in mental illness has occurred since time began and is the human condition. Creative energy being blocked by other people has severely painful and traumatic results: depression, low self-esteem and the compulsion to fail. This is an urgent problem in our addictive society because for every addict there are four people sick.

With early trauma in the sick, hostile or vacillating system a template is made of the toxic situation and the same miserable systems and cycles are repeated throughout the life of neurosis--in which one has been made sad, bad or mad. You need never feel these things again for releasing blocked energy will bring the talents of the True Self--your greatest joy in your new life.

SOCIO-BIOLOGY
Innocent Adaptation

This work is dedicated to the innocent will of God: children and animals. All animals adapt to their environments. So too man must adapt to his biological niche, his social world. This becomes his whole personality as he forgets who he is. Disease is no mystery if explained socio-biologically. Look at symptoms as simply reactions or adaptations to certain systems- -not a condition within the person. You'll open to a whole new world of the fascinating complexity of human nature. Down with psychology, up with socio-biology.

The conformist has lost his true self in order to adapt to the world--to be accepted. This puts him in instant contradiction and confusion. It is confusion and contradiction which marks the social world as people deny themselves and act by rote. All is explained by the herd matrix, the mental maze-way of the time. It is all just fashion--of thought, of ways of relating, of clothes, painting etc. all which change with the times. But the truth is timeless, transcending the follies of generations and staying fundamentally true throughout. Those who speak babble (confusion) come from Babylon but those who speak clear truth come from above--transcending all culture, family, trends, era or gender-limitations. The cosmic man is the same no matter when or where he lived. He is clear and in perfect order for God is not the author of confusion but of peace.

When genius comes whole to himself he realizes how cluttered he was with the non-essential (like things he was told to "want" and to "need"). Once whole it is austere simplicity which marks true genius--this is the seed potential at birth. Having cleared away all distractions he can now focus only on obeying God's voice inside. The opposite is neurotic "adulthood" jammed with superfluity, for the goal is the simplicity of clarity. The release of obstruction brings an automatic reversal in one's life on every level: group, mind, body. This is conversion: from blocked to clear energy. The sudden transformation from the old miserable life to the new one is called enantiodromia: everything converting to its opposite. What an excitingly unbelievable revelation: In the twinkling of an eye the sinner becomes a saint--the bottom becomes the top and the top becomes the bottom. Having dissolved old bonds keeping him down the now-realized genius attains the spiritual skies.

All Success is Attraction. Clear energy is mind energy, psychic power, will power and constancy. Since all gravity is attraction between like objects we cannot attract success when dense (fogged, distracted, hypnotized by people) while automatically the absence of obstruction attracts it all to us. Since there is no time or space (Einstein) our re-adaptation becomes an irresistible magnet to all our goals. The minute the past collapses the future has arrived. Whether you are up or down is purely a matter of blocked vs. clear energy. You choose the obstructions pulling you down. When dissolved you snap to your goal:

PEOPLE

HABIT

FOOD

This is an entirely new matrix for the life sciences: that great vitality (perfect health) is the absence of obstruction. Rid of obstruction you shoot to the stars. It's a promise: the instant switch to a new life will be felt in self, body and group. The boundaries of the old self and the bad memories of the past will melt down as if they never happened. Your self-image will suddenly improve and all social relations will switch with you on top. The subsequent release of creative energy will overwhelm you with joy.

All of your plans which would never come true will now blossom naturally having been un-jammed. You will now de-age as the release of destructive stress and tension transforms into total creative power just waiting to burst forth. Your perception and worldview dragged down to ruts have prevented progress of any kind. These rut-habits were frozen energy recycled in old channels. But when ruts are released the great new pattern emerges of a successful life.   From destructive repetition (ruts) to beautiful new patterns--that is the change you are about to see. Give up the bad associations, habits and food--then you'll release the blueprint of a gorgeous palace made impossible otherwise. Instead of losing we now win. No longer degraded by people and ruts we hit the bull's eye every time and stay on top. No more ups and downs--the saint is constant in his energy. Energy means spirit and spiritual excitement is jubilance. This ecstasy is normal!

ENERGY RELEASED

Energy is the link between the body, mind, spirit and social system and as you release bad associations and habits you will see all levels come together in an amazing new pattern. The more obstructions you release the more energy you will have, the higher in vibration you will go and the more miraculously you will see each minute come together perfectly like a jigsaw puzzle. All of the lessons people and attractions blocked by debris--the non-essential clutter in your life and diet--will now flow in naturally.   We now have the magnetism and pulling power of the most talented people in the race. Even the weakest among us can attain perfect pulling power!

WRITE A RECIPE

We are all surrounded by bothersome irritating people. We all have burdensome habits we can't seem to release. Whenever you feel down, depressed, anxious, angry or frustrated just ask yourself: who was I around, what habit was involved, what did I eat? You will surely see that one of these obstructions was involved. This is an incredibly revealing exercise which will teach you more than a library of books. Just go back one day in your life and you will find the problem obstruction that took the wind out of your sails while raining on your parade. After receiving a distressing phone call just ask: what sin, person or food preceded all of this? If it can't be found you can assume it was just a test making you your best.

Looking at life this way it can be fun to grow up--to actually use daily problems to grow up in spite of them.   If I feel attacked by someone rather than directing angry energy back I have learned to garnish self-control and look at the whole system. Inevitably I see how a relapse into an old habit--like negative thinking or associating with bad elements--attracted this toxic circumstance to me. If I ate wrong the ensuing weakness or pugnacity made me take offense where none was intended or suffer resentment for days. A pure and properly-nourished bloodstream puts me in ecstasy where none of this has effect. Always remember when down: write a recipe!

This new world-view will make you humble as you realize your own part in things, primarily your refusal to dissociate from evil elements. You must maintain humility when you attain success--by realizing that it is not you but the release from obstruction bringing you this new power: release, snap, God! You had the guts to release the bad to get to God cradling you to perfect success instead.   Humility and character will keep you there but self-congratulatory arrogance will bring your downfall. Be pure, stay sweet.

When one meets frustration he must not react as he usually does. Instead, with total self-control let this inner fire transmute to a fruit, not a fight. It is the alchemy of passion: refusing to give in (to a tantrum or habit) will create the necessary fire to make gold--the patience attracting success. Patience--the royal temperament--is the only way to muster the power to rule. Only by facing these irritations can we build this powerful fruit. It is self-control that fires frustration into freedom—that finest of all fruits. It is the lack of this control--giving in to our natural inclinations--which will take genius down to the gutter to die there. All through the centuries great genius was found dead due to a lack of self-control.

See every pugnacious person as an actor brought in by God to develop this royal quality in you as you take the throne and rise up in family or field. Only when you get to this point of maturity, humility, and spiritual perfection can you know with certainty that success is sure. And thus you can accept success, knowing you deserve it (you've taken and taken it and reacted with poise and calm) and yet you are humble, knowing how fast you can lose it!

INFINITE INTELLIGENCE

It is the physics of Einstein which lends scientific guidelines for skillful navigation of life through the eternal laws of energy and these are coterminous with the spiritual guidelines of God. Through repentance anyone can have success. Instead of betrayals and losses we now have loyalty and wins. At our wish the energy flows in to do our creative will--the will of God through us. Despite overwhelming odds we have perfect attainment. All through history sages demonstrate that less is more: one man can be a majority. Our obstructions—sin, cycles and sick systems--kept our intelligence locked in ego, a very low level of consciousness. Release the block and the very act of self-denial takes our puny minds out of the equation.   Now we can attain the Mind of God--infinite intelligence. Here is a common sequence: Has this ever happened to you?

1. The herd is working to break your mind, tame your goals and bring you down. You know it as indicated by flip-flops, sting-shots, nonverbal slights and rebuffs, whispering and harsh words and evident gossip (backstabbing and people siding against you). Whenever you enter the group they all stop talking. Your best friends are suddenly mean-spirited and it hurts.

2. Then work (inspiration) stops and you fall back into your past: your mind is now tracked into old fear, guilt and low self-esteem templates created by old systems keeping you down. Stop, yoke to God and relax. Allow time to ponder the situation by opening up to nature. Set your mind on things above--so all things below go strangely dim. It is time to give up people-worship and realize the hypnotic nature of systems that track your mind in gutter grooves.

3. Soon, in one sweeping revelation you will see: there are always an infinite number of problems but only one solution: repentance. Though the situation may not be our fault it's a test of character as repentance (elimination) allows us to meet it with power and success.

Though we may slip we intend to do right and it is the intention of the heart which prevails--and which God reads.

4. Having released the old burdens of dead habit and social infections, self-esteem alights and you are back to center: happy, healthy and holy. You are now God-centered and receive His power as the Created and the Creator properly unite. If in sin or a sick system you will not receive this power--your interest will flag and you'll lose charisma and become the "bad act." The more talented and energetic you basically are the more shameful your actions when that energy is recycled in outworn channels.

5. No matter what happened in the past, no matter how many times it happened and no matter how recently--turn from the sin, return to the right path and you are now forgiven, safe, fresh and new. Now the consequences of sin are dissolved in memory, a void is created and the reward snaps in. Reacting to bad situations in the same old ways will maintain the same patterns of lack of success, ruin, betrayal. You must now change.

Once having regained spiritual power you become an irresistible magnet to all good attractions. You now have smart, honest and enthused workers on your way to the top. This is the Truth of what Christ knew and Einstein proved:

1. It's all just energy dense to clear. Sin blocks energy down to lower dense centers. These are corrosive "traps" of desire: of flesh, power and security fears. Consciousness always goes dark and dank--hopeless despair and craving--when made dense by sin. No sin is harmless as it contains its own consequences, contained in the sin itself. Sin sends you to hell--while still on earth you fell.

2. You repent (clear) and then there is no past. The past is gone (your sins erased), the Tao moves on (memory gone, no longer habit-encased). Sin maintains bad memories: every time we give in to a craving to avoid a toxic memory, the memory is reinforced in mind--our history becomes more inflamed and distorted. Repentance smashes through this magnified holocaust to bring fond memories of the past--the slate is wiped clean in the erasure of sin. It was only our sins which carried the past around to beat us up.

3. All gravity is attraction. Having released obstruction (the past has collapsed) the future has arrived (an overnight success). If adversity merely bend a man, it only made him stronger (attractive to all-good, repelling all-bad). Einstein proved that gravity falls towards (rather than down) things of like affinity. The Law of Affinity is: things of like tone vibrate together. We attract what we are, not what we say we are. If in sin, we automatically attract evil elements and repel the good. If pure we repel the bad and snap into the good in what seems like a pure accident. This force-filled law cannot be changed!

It's fun to be clear and clean--to be pure is to be fast, quick, ecstatic. This is the reality God meant for man, not heaviness and despair. A closer look at the three obstructions will compare the difference--their a drag (on perception), a jam (of creative energy waiting to burst through) and a snag (in your work).

SYSTEMS

The human group is tribalistic--held together by enforced conformity which punishes non-conformity and uniqueness. 85% of rejection is through nonverbal gestures of which one is unaware--though it registers subconsciously and hurts physically. The only way to conform is to block energy: mal-adapt and live by rote. This dulled adaptation creates mediocrity. In groups we compete through established rules based only on tradition, precedent or (in the case of dysfunctional systems) the fears and anxieties of the dominant. Our uniqueness--our biological striving to be and become our highest potential is blocked, our spirit choked.

THE BOX MIND

The mental adaptation is the box mind. Box thinking is the mentality of the crowd: it sees statistics as the truth, stereotypes as good and right, and group consensus as "morality". The box mind is a mindless clone that chooses not to be independent. The box thinker is legalistic and concerned only with appearance, bringing harshness to the personality. He may be in total agreement with you and flip-flop suddenly when getting with another box thinker. Consistency in thought—trustworthiness--only comes with true independence and strength of conviction which the box thinker lost long ago. To buttress up strength he relies on bloat, boasting and backstabbing to gain approval.

A genius growing up in this atmosphere has much fodder to work with as he can use it to maximize his strength in resistance. If he can see it this way he can succeed greatly. Turning lemons into lemon-aid will turn the most senseless tragedies into glorious triumphs of never-before-seen masterpieces on earth. Go for it. Learn to thank God for all obstructions for the more the obstruction the greater the reward for coming through it. It is very difficult to overcome--become impervious to--the harshness of these legalistic systems. Cruel put-downs are a way of maintaining the status quo-with one up, the other down. Sting-shots and flip-flops--the indicators of a sick system--are the ways the dominant maintain it. Cruelty becomes embedded as a trigger to incur anxiety and maintain the bad identity of the misfit and the system set-up. If you threw tantrums at these triggers your new powerful life begins the minute you don't. This is such a powerful change that the system erupts and if you can maintain your poise you'll end up on top. Make gold at the scapegoat system and enantiodromia can now occur as everything converts to its opposite. Now the top becomes the bottom and the bottom becomes the top. Hah! the scapegoat system stumbling block has now become your stepping stone into success.

STUMBLING BLOCK BECOMES STEPPING STONE
Scapegoat Systems

Genius is created in problematic soil but flourishes only in non-problematic soil (having seen the hypnotic trance he was under in the system). Had he stayed blind he would never have been able to see the gem he was meant to be. He must transcend the family system to become whole--only then can the others (the covertly sick) recover too. To evoke awareness one should know how the system operates:

Human systems block through conformity and competition. Fear--not love--prevails as one must become hyper-alert to social cues not creative ones. As he adapts to the moods of others he becomes entangled—contaminated--by their own illness. This makes him even more hyper-alert to--entirely focused on--the others until he becomes one with them.   Insofar as he stays involved he remains created--and sickened--by the system.   Self-control--not reacting no matter what--will smash through memory and the tendency to tantrum while creating a whole new authentic identity in us. This non-reaction makes us instantly new people: the refusal to play releases the true self and the unique genius therein. Don't forget--we identify ourselves by how others see us--and in that system that has been bad (not in God's image).

These sick systems are steeped in identity crisis. Since all identity is relational---how we see ourselves against the background of others--the members must keep the patient down to maintain their own identity intact. If the genius is a scapegoat nothing he can do or say will change the negative perceptions people have of him--his stigma. To accept his true identity would put theirs in jeopardy so those on top don't want to revert—by truly seeing the squirt. But if the would-be genius can learn to not react, fast and wait so enantiodromia--the big shift with him on top—can occur, the world will call him "sir" and his foes will become a blur.

THE PSYCHOLOGY OF DIAGNOSTICIANS
Labeling Theory

This need for the sick system to maintain its identity of being "good", "nice", "considerate" or "loving" against the backdrop of his badness or madness is a common tragedy in the medical/care-giving professions.   Often an insecure therapist who may experience competitive or envious feelings with the female "patient' may link with the system—like the two jealous older sisters--to "put her down." Both the professional and the family may be unaware of the abuse of power for the sake of their own identity. Let's take an example of an insecure female physician (very few people are truly secure) who officiously gets involved in family problems to feel superior to the patient towards whom she feels competitive ("there is no house big enough for two women." Female competition is evident in several other species like dogs).

Throughout the literature on systems theory (on schizophrenia, alcoholism, anorexia and AA: anorexic-alcoholism) we see examples of this collusion between the sick family and insecure therapist. An weak male caregiver may be sexist-- threatened by a strong female patient whom he wants to "put in her place." He will often link with the toxic family against her, jealous of her "arrogant" force of will. It is naïve to think that just because one wears a professional label he/she is devoid of such human characteristics, for jealousy is the biggest emotion in the human race! Championship training is learning how to deal with thugs assaulting and accusing the ace.

As you can see the nightmare of human systems is bigger than the family unit. The system is nonsummative: the whole is bigger than the sum of its parts. If the scapegoat doesn't stand up with strength (rather than lay down with weakness) he may be hounded to his death or worse-- institutionalized. There are multitudes of rare genius never heard from again as the very differences defining their rare aptitude gets them locked up for life. Genius who overcomes is rare--many die of suicide or drugs in response to the painful plight of persecutory put-downs. The soon-skeptical stigmatized soul sees everyone as having the loyalty of a rattlesnake. The box mind--the group mind, the devil's crowd--was most evident in Nazi Germany. Many Germans had Jews as friends but overnight the Jewish reality turned black as images changed. People are controlled by agreed-upon images, not their own perception. Social irascibility and cruelty is not peculiar to the Germans but is evident in all tribes and cultures to different degrees. It is human nature which has the capacity for both soaring heights and devastating lows. Man's quest for identity--to feel superior--has no bounds in human pounds!

RECAP: CONTRADICTION AND CULTURE

1. It is mixed signals that mark the social world. Needing approval man is constantly focused on the social reality leaving no time, energy or receptivity to the higher creative. In genius this loss brings low self-esteem and more co-dependence on the sick system which continues to block his energy and hold him down.

2. The "herd" is not a person but a mentality. Through constant conformity and feedback it dances in perfect synchrony as if to a drum. This induces a trance state where no matter what "all seems normal." Absurdity is seen as "normal" simply because it is prevalent. Dancing in perfect step to an absurd but taken-for-granted-as-normal-tune (called social "morality") the herd reacts harshly to genius "deviancy" to the dance.

3. Thus genius is lost early in life. Why? Because man's quest to belong is that strong. He may boast of his mental independence but watch closely while he foolishly marches in step with the current line. True genius cannot conform to time and place--fad or fashion--but is fundamental: a rare timeless achievement.

2

GENIUS MUST GET UP

Repent, Detach Disaster and No Longer be Cheap

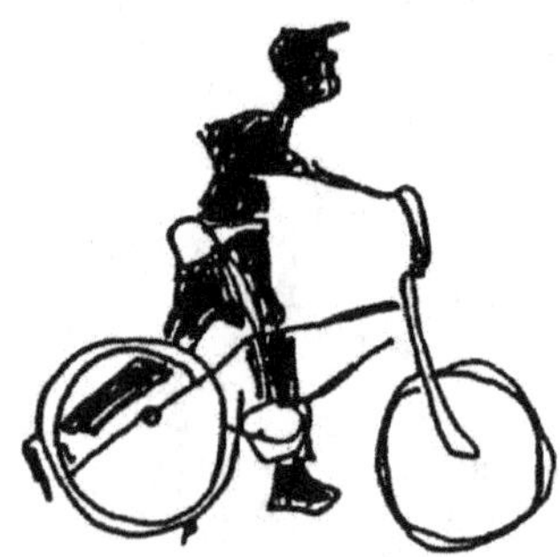

People want to tell you how to live. That's a fact--if one cannot see it he's so "well-adapted" he's lost the vision of freedom. Genius must be free in order to realize his destiny of due recognition and remuneration. This means free of invading elements or the expectation to socially adapt. Realized genius is simply someone who has learned to manage human relations--to carve out his way letting no one dissuade. Old style psychology obtusely tells the client what he should want and how he should adapt to society. Jungian psychology in contrast elicits from the patient what he wants and gives him the tools to solve all other questions through his own inner journey.

The most important word genius must learn is "NO." The world is filled with miserable YES people doing what they don't want just to gain approval. Look around to those you meet-- do you sense a desolate darkness, a watered-down wasteland? That's the face of a yes-man. He's filled with frustration but has adapted against his true wishes for so many years he doesn't realize it. He becomes passive-aggressive--a "nice guy" who shows his anger by being late, not calling, standing you up etc. Frustration always leads to aggression and it will come out sooner or later on the weakest elements around.

We are a generation who have perfected phoniness, serving another God--the social world--who will kills us. Those who care what others think have lost all direction in life, as their mood changes with whomever was last spoken to or what someone "said." A moody person is an outer-directed person and the outer-directed become moody as substances and people invade the temple and mind. If you're going nowhere any road will take you there. As he becomes unknowingly contaminated he can no longer distinguish between his thoughts and the group's. Extreme outer direction was the Nazi campaign as social hypnotism justified evil or anorexogenic systems where the group mind substitutes for "leader."

NOSY OLD PSYCHOLOGY

Old psychology officiously objects to the inner journey as it cannot be controlled or talked to. It mysteriously belongs to the person alone and does not abide outside interference. This the "psyche pro" cannot stand. He wants you to compete with him on his turf--your insistence to be alone within your boundaries means he's lost for his theories and curiosities cannot go there. If one wants to stay home so his adaptive energy can be focused on the project at hand society rebels for it looks like social anxiety or "missing out" on what they have to offer. If a genius is not strong enough to stave off aggression from family, neighbors etc. he could easily find himself sided against and then even institutionalized. Lone non-social females in Nazi Germany were often put in concentration camps--on no other evidence than the dossiers of suspicious neighbors. One needs strength to forge ahead so the unique blueprint can evolve on its own accord. Learning how to deal with people and their coercions is the pivotal point determining the rise or the fall of genius.

RELEASING OBSTRUCTION
Genius is simple like a child

Disease and aging come from obstruction. Freedom and de-aging come from elimination. Genius must be an ageless child: creative, clean, carefree. Like Einstein he must be "mild, saintly and sober." This ageless state comes from released obstruction. Once clean and clear he becomes more creative with each decade up until the moment of death and continues to peel back to the birth symbol, the unspoiled seed potential of who he is. What freedom! How sad to be blocked by nosy do-gooders whose "concern" could destroy a destiny. The roadmap to the power of real royal reign is human management and trusting only God.

All obstruction is just useless baggage to be eliminated for progress to continue. The body/mind is a flexible energy field. When clear we feel ecstatic as energy goes through us finding its true mark in the world. Mental contamination--social infection--chokes talent, darkens the aura and denses the field. It completely clouds creative clout--the charisma which would win every time. When happy we have a transparent glow. When clogged or contaminated we are opaque--a dead dry brick--as the eyes glaze over. If you've ever been held down you may remember the relief of separation. That's the feeling of Self-Return!

After being so belittled, misquoted and told what to feel, want and think it will feel so good to just avoid.

Clear (unobstructed) we actually vibrate with a delightful electrical sensation. As energy flows our psychology--where we block--determines how our body looks as well as all else. For example, bio-energetically when women block (or allow others to block) their self-expression that energy stops at the waist and the hips and thighs bulge. But if clear the body streamlines and there is a mysterious undercurrent that magnetizes and heals those we meet in a contagion of enlightenment. The mind fizzles with creative thought and joy. But if again blocked through sin or people we miss the mark and relapse into the "bad act" or even dumber mistakes. The synapses are caulked so creative energy warps in error and embarrassment.

People and habits drain energy. Without ecstatic jubilance there can be no champion, but with repentance brings an explosive creative release into a brand new life. In an instant the miseries are gone, the old cycle ends just as the new one begins. Since it was people and habits which maintained bad memories the past and its awful recall are gone forever and jubilance (true freedom) is here.

GENIUS IS PURE
Transcending Cultural Neuroses (The Herd)

The righteous are powerful, the sinners are weak. The public speaker whose private life is impure will bore or irritate the audience--the anointing of God won't be there and the extreme self-consciousness coming from sin will destroy his talent. Clothes, looks, fame and fortune won't work--its only the power of anointed genius which speaks to the collective unconscious. Only this evokes subconscious analogies bringing true insight and change. What happens in our private lives has everything to do with our public life.

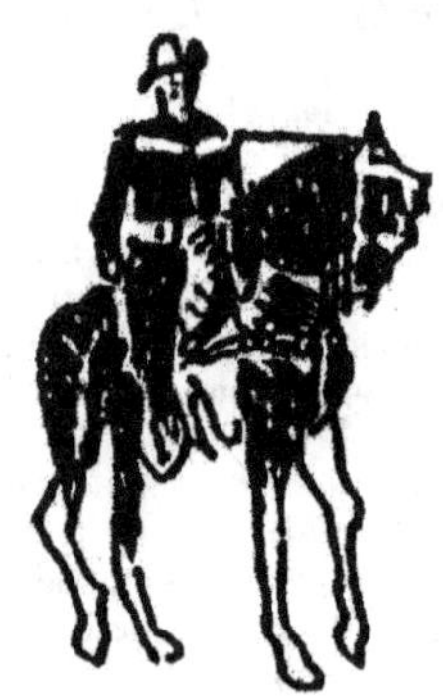

One must have nothing to do with the secular world. Since it is opposite to the True Self it will always infect with low self-esteem. Are you young or old? Male or female? Rich or poor? A fit or a misfit? These dichotomies and stereotypes are the cultural neurosis, the herd. For everyone these will trigger intense self-doubt and fear at some point in life. Whenever you feel doubt, fear or low self-esteem check the environment--did someone bring the herd in? Sanctify your home (your power-base and insulation from the world) and make it your monastery: now join the spirit of victory.

SYSTEMS THEORY AND GENIUS

At first insanity is a mal-adaptation to a particular culture or system. Later it is triggered interactionally. Someone can be normal when alone but sick when involved due to flimsy boundaries. These are the hypersensitives easily hurt by contradictions, manipulations and the leveling processes that keep people "ordinary." The mature genius has learned how to manage people who want to manage him and resolving these boundary disputes are the mainstay of his talent. The social mechanisms which make you conform--the glue of groups, the tribal instinct--are taken-for-granted as "normal" by less sensitives who can "get along with people" or "pass go." The current line of thought--the herd mentality--is assumed to be truth or the way the world "works." Groupies demand we see reality that way--a severe invasion of boundaries and the reason genius secludes in his own niche: to avoid misjudgment and strife.

TWO MAL-ADAPTANTS

The herd makes two kinds of people sick: the anxious-misfit-turned-conformist and the herd member who has become dull, dimmed and ordinary from so much adaptation. He's worn the mask for so long he's a stranger to his True Self. Only the people living with him know who he really is--what he has become, this split being. Come home--leave the split, go to spirit. Both the misfit and the conformist are lost: the would-be genius nervously trying to belong and the jaded dull groupie. Only the True Self sits in the light, the pure symbol God designed and all else is dark. Both types mal-adapt to the mixed signals in society and in both cases energy is blocked and inner reality impoverished. At one time the great genius Beethoven lived in a small town filled with small-minded hate for him. Children would mock and beat him up as he walked by. He could not distinguish between his reality and their projections so he took it all on and became a derelict in his appearance (but simultaneously wrote his greatest concerts in his flat). Its very hard not to take on the projections of others. The fact that Beethoven did great work in spite of it all was a mark of his inner strength. But most mature genius learns to insulate from even the possibility of taking it on, for guarding the anointing of the creative spirit is the utmost concern! This is true humility--for he knows how easily he can lose that power.

It is the most energetically creative who become the worst when dropping self to adapt to society. If we clamp down on self to guard against misjudgment our behavior is "warped" as every thing is said and done for the wrong reasons. True genius comes from the heart fresh or it warps in error. Can he learn to ignore harsh hostility and just do his work? For that is his only protection--staying high above the multitudes. He fights--he loses. For most this means staying alone until success which is now able to occur. Don't forget--mediocrity brings confirmation while true genius brings massive opposition particularly in these days of brainless entertainment and a severely dumbed-down public school system. He cannot forbear a vulgar prostitution of talent for true genius is good taste while immaturity degrades with vulgarity (to get approval of the mindless mob). It's hard to watch the gross and compromising get acceptance while the fine and excellent truth is shunned!

UNIQUE GENIUS BRINGS REJECTION

Creativity is limited by anything which channels or constrains it. Genius cannot be burdened with social inhibitions necessary to tow the line. He cannot "fit" the social dance for on every level of the hierarchy--eighty-five percent of which is nonverbal--he is disqualified. From eye-blinks to posture he's a misfit: too different, odd and socially deviant. Others get used to the ordinary, the sameness of most people and so may react vehemently to these differences. The genius is sensitive to this harshness and rejection and so may try to gain social favor by "learning" belonging styles. Being of the same culture he knows how people like himself are viewed and tries everything to adapt, to conform, to banish his hideous stigma. But the more he tries to gain social favor the more hideous he becomes--so far removed from the rich spontaneity of the True Self. The more dense the herd (limiting, stereotypic, non-creative) the more stifling.

The unique genius deserving of fame creates shame instead If he needs social approval which punishes the unique. Energy is either turned outward to creative self-expression or inward to creative self-destruction. Because it often mal-adapts through addiction--thus losing it's talent as well as it's sanity--true genius is rare. It is killed off early either by the leveling processes of the herd or by addictive mal-adaptations. The herd mentality can be so brutal that successful methods of avoiding social anxiety can be very addicting. The exhaustion from overcoming obstacles to selfhood often ends in death through suicide or drugs. The mundane herd reality--the obstacles to creativity and the "ordinarization" of the person--is overwhelming to the sensitive who finds he can only create his own personal reality in the face of it through mind-altering chemicals. As he becomes progressively more dependent his solitude ends in death. Lost genius is the greatest casualty of the mundane!

GENIUS POTENTIAL LIES DORMANT

Genius is everyone's birthright but it is only a dormant potential--a "surplus potential developed in problems areas." It is developed from overcoming obstacles after which it naturally blossoms into maturity. All animals have seed potentials and unique genius is ours. Genius is born of obstructive obstacles but matures only through moral purification--by eliminating the addictive coping devices dealing with ridicule, rejection and necessary reclusion. This feeling of being a stranger in a strange land, the gut feeling of being abandoned and lost is a result of his separation from the True Self, not just society.

Via everyday face-to-face interactions original behaviors have been punished in the family, the social network and by the public. Nonverbal slights and rebuffs may not be consciously acknowledged but underground the gut and heart churns shame, fear and grief.   Little does the genius realize he may be far superior to the others--who have long since stunted their growth in order to belong--to maintain dependency in fear of loneliness. Hyper-sensitives show a "genius gene": hyper-sensitivity to contradiction. This leads them to great breakthroughs in the arts and sciences--landmark works which smash through silly precedents and myths. But this sensitivity also means they end up alone--in a desire for sweet saintly solitude.

RISING THROUGH RECTITUDE

To gain sufficient force to transcend the power of social constraints the genius must have self-assurance and certitude of Who He Is and that He Is Right. Then he can go fast forward to perfect success--world revolution in his field. This kind of self-assured certitude only comes from moral rectitude--of knowing he is right. The same energy plunging to shame becomes fame as the worst becomes the best in this transformation of energy. This is the fine art of energy transmutation: By giving up social needs and secluding and then repenting the aspirant purifies his energy and insulates his mind against mental contamination and manipulation. He takes his eyes off the herd and puts them on work and world. What a glorious relief--now things are easy and joyous as he attracts admirers to team his masterpiece.

Life has many seasons. One season is destroyed by people and vices used to dull the pain of life, but in a later season one separates from these wasteful sins and associations and sanctifies his life instead. Now free he can just do his work for the world. Refocused and recharged he transcends social approval and gains real world recognition.   The very behaviors bringing ridicule in early life become the means, talents and tools of Victory. Though genius is born in problematic soil it flourishes only in non-problematic soil: in eliminating the nosy busybodies he comes to maturity, out of obscurity.

SOCIETY IS SENSELESS
Silly Social Sickness

We can only make sense of society by realizing it makes no sense. Then wisdom arrives. Note the following Bible passages: "Only he who hateth the world shall gain eternal life....they love only their own--the others they despise...they hated me before they hated you...only God is good." Or as Jesus said to the church leaders, priests and scribes (who later killed him): "Pharisees, hypocrites. You're outside is beautiful but inside you are dead men's bones and all uncleanliness...all your doings are to be seen of men." Jesus hated hypocrisy the most. Insanity comes from adapting to hypocrisy by going blind to it. Once we become blind to it we are it!

The herd is the perversion of tribalism, the leveling process destroying creative action and growth. It's an automatic rejection of the novel, the unique, and so genius learns to expect and avoid harshness. If genius can learn to insulate to develop on his own accord, his talents and skills can evolve through purity until His Time Has Come. Otherwise genius dies early from addictions-to-cope with the constant stress of misjudgment. Genius is the unique flowering of the very peculiarities the world puts down. Early life is smashed in collision with the world forces that disdain these differences. If he accepts their view the addictive devices become traps of ruin. Genius doesn't fit so must get strong to make a way or break a path. He is meant to make a peculiar difference and amazing new dent as God's "peculiar treasure" and True Delight. The preparation is overcoming obstacles, the reward is world success and justified remuneration. Genius is evoked and evolves in the problem—but only gets the prize by overcoming the problem.

No first-class soldier gets entangled in the enemy's ways and traditions. We are entangled! There's a perfect path for each man but we can't get to it roped to the stake of society--or the past. We must live a holy life--meaning a separated life. To prosperously hum along in our own stream Jesus said "come out from amongst them [separate] and I shall give you great favor." To overcome the powerful world constraints to genius we must strengthen a vessel free of all doubt by clearing out these deadening blocks:

MOOD SWINGS

The dense mal-adaptor has constant mood swings covered over by a social image to appear constant. The inner conflict between who he is and who he says he is creates vicious changes of mood and cruel--though "polite"--explosions onto other people. These explosions are bio-devices to relieve stress and are also masked through an image of "niceness" ("polite cruelties"). It is these contradictions which drive genius mad. This contradictory matrix and the resulting insanity mark the crowded conditions of the modern (non-natural) world of man. If in fear we let social anxiety hitch us up to others we lose our own reality where the bliss is and then wonder "why am I always so tired?" What holds us down? Other people. When down look only to future glory--persist on the inner journey to the Self and trust only God.

You can be having a wonderful day moving point-to-point in your own little cornucopia—puttering, pondering, petting your animals, playfully creating. Then someone arrives and debates against your life. You've suddenly gone from light to dark. Now you've experienced what the Indians did with the incursion of legalistic dogmas or tyrannical "shoulds." You've not yet learned to simply nip it in the bud: "I don't want to debate--live and let live." Then you could have stayed happily bathed in light. Instead you "got involved" on their level, went dense and woke up irritable. Stand strong! If not strong enough to block the blockers you'll mal-adapt through sin.

ZVENGALI SYSTEMS
Happy Release Through "No"

When a strong person is even subtly or politely insulted he says "NO" and moves away from the interaction. A weak person--made dense by previous systems--is actually hooked to the toxic dominance. The unfinished business from the past compels him to work to change the rejection or rebuff. The rejecter looms large as he needs his approval more. He keeps himself down at this point by looking up to people rather than God. Although people were his problem he becomes a people-worshipper. And thus he is a perfect complement to the Zvengali who keeps self-esteem low to maintain the relationship. His biggest problem is asking for advice when only God's advice matters! Unsuitable advice--people's advice--will never hit the mark for God's ways are higher than man's and the genius blueprint can never be mapped out or predicted by another.

Self-esteem is the only way to illumination and reaching the goal—it's an ego-less life just between you and God. It's this divine relationship which gives you self-esteem--not a person, lest a Zvengali relationship easily develop. Self-esteem can't be faked for the false will always fail. It's this point of purity that precedes success. If total aloneness brings panic and one calls or slips (into bad) the gold ring is lost again, perhaps for good. Don't worry if old systems leave your scene--your new growth disrupts their comfort zone! And asking for their advice is a sure sign you're "not there" yet. By refusing entanglement in the world and its values you're offering yourself to God. "Be not conformed--be ye transformed." Overcome the world by going beyond it, to walk with God as you work and win. Let Him get a hold of your whole mind so your life proves what is good. Leave nothing out as you relate to Him. God's will is the best for you, your will is mediocre and the will and advice of other people is no-where.

WORLD SPLITS IN TWO

The world explodes into two potentialities: a spiraling down to the same old ruts or a new heaven on earth through the agency of true genius-now-revealed. One must decide between world and God--to go back down or be catapulted up. The natural unfolding of the universe is like cells which always divide between higher consciousness and those choosing to stay (in the status quo). The earth is split between the old and the new. The old won't realize anything but its own chaos and pain while you will have instantaneous ascendance just by repentance and regaining the anointing. Do you have the courage to just trust God and let all the old go or stay down and listen to your "friends"? There is no more time to vacillate from momentary enlightenment to the doldrums. You must now stay steady. Don't be surprised as the world rips away from you--God wants you to heal so deal with present pain by looking ahead: think futuristically.

EARLY REJECTIONS

Very few geniuses have not suffered early rejection. With this background they wear their peculiarity on their sleeve: Tremendous guilt and shame remains-"maybe I am bad, a criminal, too-sad, perhaps mad..." He shuts down emotionally and wears the armor of a porcupine. It doesn't help to tell the victim: "your early rejection is a sign of their inability to love rather than your unlovability." After early rejection the social order becomes more important to him than what he wants as the rejection is unfinished business seeking social correction. Instead truly correct it through the development of talent, forgetting social approval and seeking God's instead.

LIBERTY

The problem of early rejection is magnified when in order to belong we banish our own liberty--which could enlighten the world. Staying alone to evolve and prepare is very important to the world! The result of self-work is charm and taste--two traits very lacking in everyday man who mistakenly thinks the liberty to be is actually the liberty to sin. Thinking he is "liberated" he substitutes lust-enslavement for true independence. Peace-liberty-enlightenment only comes by being your True Self revealed in purity. When God's spirit is refracted to the social--which occurs in many churches--there is much trouble as genius (intended as the true reflection of God) erodes.

The statue of "liberty" is not a symbol of domination but of power! Every human being can have victory as a genius child of God when free of bondage. All other illusions of "liberty" are lies. Get free and just do your work in happy harmony, not the pain of pettiness. This revival looks forward to the harvest, the ultimate goal of the changes of spring--as Genius Gets Up Again. Oh lukewarm and lonely genius--revival restores! Just set your mind on things above so that things below go strangely dim. Forget your fair-weather friends--for "happy is the man whose mind is stayed on Him." Then happy will be your work hours as you seek the unsought and teach the untaught. Like a lightening flash creative insight will come forth to dent the earth--the searing light of God's truth in your work. Along with hard work and perseverance you will have your Great Reward: here on earth, and soon.

ORDER IN SOLITUDE
The higher the boundaries the more orderly.

Without God isolation can be more terrible than sleeping on ice. If in sin it suffocates with loneliness and creates insanity. But with purity-in-God it's exhilarating as you appreciate beauty as never before. Reveling in freedom the mind escapes time and distance. A fine thing to feel the mind go voyaging through space! This mind transport blows out all the circuits of early rejection. Now just stay put, fast and avoid all old sins and systems. If it's only the fast which brings on this consciousness then you must fast consistently. Solitude will change your life so you can come back freshly endowed with new powers and make your amazing new dent. The older family scapegoat said "suddenly all my persecutors were finally gone. I couldn't believe how good I felt. The lifelong block dissolved I instantly attracted world success for the things I had worked for all my life."

In solitude (liberty) new schemes are developed to increase the content of the minutes and hours. By doing things systematically the biggest variety of sensory input is provided and the mind soon becomes universally receptive--everywhere at all times. As this fascinating journey continues to increase we cannot tolerate too-much social stimulation and all work habits and isolation are geared to keep stable the brain's arousal. Suddenly our lives go from casual to formal: no more drop-ins, just appointments. It's a gold mine only in purity--for if twisted in sin we are separated from God (total darkness). and automatically fall in with lower associates. Work to please God, not people.

TO SOAR:

Make peace with your family and all toxic templates. Reject all agitators--as denial lifts you'll see them all around. Reject the bars and reach for the stars. Instead of praying to God to "make something happen" you must ask: "where from? The outer world? It only dulls." Just pray and wait for happenings inside---then the outer world becomes your oyster.

3

BAD FAITH OR FULLNESS?

Faith in Abusers or Ecstasy?

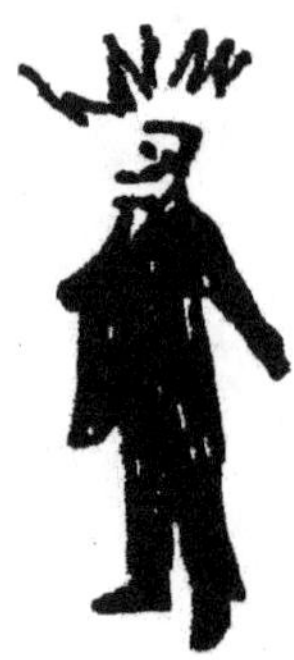

You can either have fullness of experience--each moment vivid rich perception of the universe, or bad faith--faith in a hurtful or useless person, but you cannot have both. As soon as you put your faith in the wrong person you'll have lost your miraculous perception and be dragged down to bland, boring, petty, mean, shallow and mundane reality. Watch who you put your faith in. Simply put, watch who you associate with--because the influence is there with the mere contact. The shark knows this: his sequence is contact, influence, conquest! The conquest is over your mind which ceases to be a lovely garden and starry night and starts being a scene from hell. In those times you can make a wrong decision which will degrade your life for decades. Dissociating with lower elements is the name of the fame game at this point--you must separate in order to re-connect to the powers that be in your field.

Do you think that just because someone is popular and accepted that you should put your faith in them? Don't kid yourself, for the opposite is true. Falling into the popular groove they are constantly out of grace and will only misadvise you on what you should do. Look back--were not all of the past tragedies due to some involvement or influence with other people? It's scary to realize this but incredibly beneficial. Thinking most people are "nice" is very stupid--stay alert to subtle influences tearing you down.

The wrong faith object will inspire fear in you. This fear is your inner instinct crying out against possible destruction--its your solar plexus indicating a sense of powerlessness. The Bible says "faith in an unstable man is like living on quicksand." Though you may be dulling your instincts to avoid this recognition your insides are distressed from what you know down deep. You must listen to what your body is telling you--are you stuffing or drinking down your fear-recognitions?

You must now become aware of and question your associates. Because I tell you truth--you will never go anywhere if you stay in that situation for you need silence to succeed and this present situation is noise—games. Above all else keep chatterers (or those using you for entertainment) at bay for these are energy thieves. You must cut them loose for the time is late. Many of your sins are just coping devices to adapt to these people--your environment. Man is an adaptive animal--and the mal-adaptation to dense environments is exhaustion. Exhaustion is the result of oppression--from letting inferior people worm their way in.

Because these dense environments are characterized by sterile dynasties and petty competition they contaminate and restrict your creativity. They are based on a whole other set of rules that you want no part of. Your destiny will only unfold through your own genius which acts point-to-point without a map or a plan. Only silence allows your focus on what to do next. Remember it's the weak who talk too much. They cannot understand why you'd rather think than talk. Let them go. Even if you have to live with animals at least you'll get your work done. It will be effortless--with holy spirit ease--if you can separate and establish your own reality with God. Only there do you get the divine design of each moment, the grand culmination of which is total success in your field. You've been resurrected from the dead, a case of beauty from ashes.

THE DEVIL'S CROWD

The Devil's Crowd is politically correct. They tow the line: they think and say whatever's "popular". But it's only the tyranny of the group that wants you to think you're the one who's down and hopeless. For a long time you've been trying to prove yourself which only allowed them to keep you down more due to your guilt and their disapproval. You must learn to say "I refuse to deal with your projections and cannot talk again."   To overcome this subtle yet pervasive obstacle, become assertive. The dominator adapted to your docility so look them in the eye, say "no" and never think of these old networks again. Once eliminated your attractive powers will link to success. Just be right so no more memories, habits or systems can take hold.

As long as you're never around gossip can't hurt you--you're just a name or label. You've grown weary in your one-down state so declare independence and bid them good-bye. When you're out of the system there's nothing they can do, so keep thinking when down: "my aura has been contaminated and infected. Soon I'll be better, then the best. I now release this system and transcend to my world talent." In regards to these particular people the "case is closed." If upon waking up to the abuse you find yourself without friends, great--now you'll be with God, the highest. God knows your great future--this present situation is part of your training. It's heartbreaking dealing with people when coming into your own talents-

-a free world--but just remember this: jealousy is their incentive! People attempt to make you feel small to avoid them feeling that way when you get so big!

TWO   CHOICES

We have a choice: Faith in wrong people (bad faith) or the experience of true fullness. Bad faith brings depression while recognition of the truth about people brings recovery into fullness. You can't have both. There's no happiness with bad faith as the contradictions are a cancer to the subconscious. When the tension of denial is gone you're back in the Kingdom: your center, your home. Acceptance reached brings your reversal: you're now in a joyful light so just accept the truth and your life will change suddenly. These people putting painful projections all over you care nothing for your joy. Bad faith in useless people is maintained through denial resulting in dimmed experience, flagged interest, dulled eyes and dense brain--you no longer "cherish the day." Everything forced unconscious makes us dense: anytime we deny the obvious the whole project dims. Through your relationship alone the wrong person can degrade your reality--the hard-won bud of genius. This beautiful seed is smashed by the carnal, the vulgar and the indifferent. Once the light goes out due to relationship, bad habits and memories the creative process is ruined. True pleasure is blocked from tension. Release prideful people and pastimes and you'll find fullness: ecstasy in life.

GROUP ENMESHMENT
Cunning competition

We lose self when enmeshed in groups to which we must drop parts of self to adapt. We should be moving to a more independent reality, not a more enmeshed one. The most extreme example of independence is the discoverer who always splits from the majority view. He must be strong and pure to silently maintain his view which "everyone knows is false". Such high boundaries is an achievement and an absolute must for success to occur, for separation precedes completion. Another example is the anorexic who was undifferentiated from the family system in youth so now compensates by taking the opposite track in maturity--total reclusion.   After many mishaps she learns that petty competition and jealousies are instantly dissolved with her total inaccessibility. To guard against relapse she guards her mind and selects all that gets in her body, mind and environment. Whereas she was a "blank slate" for others projections she now becomes warm steel--cordial but firm, impervious to influences. She jealously guards who's around for it is "contact, influence, conquest."

We know that children love non-competitive games the most--it is independence that brings full self-expression. The happiest cultures are non-competitive and true genius competes with no one--that talent is unique and in its own stream there is no competition. Competitive left-brain groups ruin genius. The rare overcomer avoids such and never compares himself to anyone--this usually means staying on his own turf.

YOUR   PRIVATE   CASTLE

CHAMPION GUIDES

Your essence is your private castle for nothing else compares. To be home-centered is to be self-centered—this is good. If your home doesn't reflect you, you lack center and are owned by society. When people lack a center their home is often in shambles while they spend time away. You must regain your center to feel that wonderful joy of knowing the you as distinguished from the masses. The non-competitive atmosphere of your home transcends time and space. So become inaccessible, choose your experience, make your home reflect your personality and never adapt again! From now on you choose all as you simultaneously seclude. Love your little niche, filling time with solitary pursuits to establish your own separate reality. Through the inner journey you gain the discernment and high boundaries defining True Royalty.

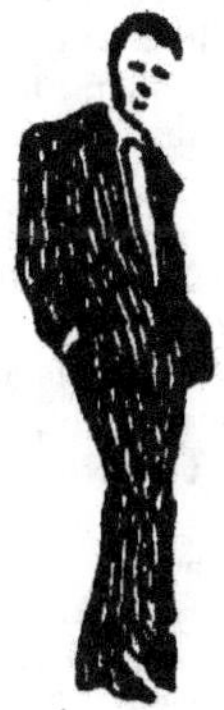

SCIENCE OF SILENCE
Vs. Codependency

If one is right, then silence is the most perfect way to deal with resistance. No one expects anything from the rightly inaccessible! If your way is best then be that silent stream of refreshment, for people who need you as teacher. Until one's time has come, fighting resistance will only tear him down. But surety, silence and seclusion will manage new attractions and prevent falling victim again. In most groups loyalty and protection take precedence over autonomy and self-realization--and so they will always side against the Great. In groups denial of self combined with mutual consideration are far more esteemed than the expression of Self. But for the genius there is sanctity to separation and seclusion--until the time comes to express and catalyze the race: to be the genius in the field. The opposite to this release into cosmic freedom is the horrors of codependency:

Bad faith is really about co-dependency where the dominant one maintains his superior identity by "helping" or "advising" others--and then getting angry when they don't obey or go their own way. Such anger inspires fear which leads to more bad faith and lost fullness. Put your faith where it belongs--in your own stream and instincts for then your own moments will be protected by God. As you get strong the dominant will spread a net to trap you but he will fall into it. Rather than resisting his competitive strivings it is patient perseverance in one's own stream which breaks the false power of codependency. "Holy" means separate--like God. To be holy is to be separate.   Because God is separate, holy is removed from the ordinary. The highest form of religious experience is to reflect and imitate the divine--so separate and insulate and God will shine through your talents now unfolding. This period of "ecstatic rest" is your last phase. For new royalty, rest precedes rule.

CRUEL PEOPLE

My favorite social theorist is Vernon Howard whose theories of human nature are priceless. When I read his work on "ways to escape cruel people" my life came together as the hypnotic spell of various systems dissolved. I finally saw the mixed signals that kept me down. It was shocking because I always felt blame and shame but could not see the set-up as spectator. "Cruel people" is a little jewel revealing those human cruelties so you may shake loose from the denial of bad faith.

Every detachment from fruitless destructive relationships brings explosion into new wonderlands. Once the grieving is complete a brand new life opens up. The release is as elevating as a long fast which brings total transformation. One's "self" has been defined against these grounds, so detach and now the universe and God--the lovely moment--defines you. The wonderful release is ineffable! The past's heartbreak of violence and indifference dissolves to joy in the glorious opening after the painful control. Cruelty is usually too subtle, silent and insidious to see and thus we seldom hear about it. We only hear of "love" and "goodness"--the masks we're told to wear, while cruelty is rarely mentioned (let alone detailed) because as a sinister force it prevents its own exposure. But the shocking facts will liberate you with perfect protection so learn them well as most all cruelty is unnoticed as it happens too often and fast for the mind to register. It all adds up to thousands of pains: a broken promise or plan, being stood up or kept waiting, gossip-called-concern, a perverse triangle or secret alliance, the hostile stare, the sarcastic contemptuous remark, dangerous advice, a "casual" misjudgment or false advertising.

There is active cruelty (hateful insults), then the passive cruelty of witnessing and allowing it to occur--like a mother who won't defend her children against an abusive husband. It's an invisible empire with millions of unaware humans constantly punished by their own ignorance. For though unaware it registers deep resulting in addictions to avoid anxiety— it's the cause of a pervasive anger whose source remains hidden. It's the fear of facing its vastness that prevents escape.   Our denial keeps us hooked to the cruel effects while awareness though painful gives perfect protection and prevention of any more hurt. It does not leave by ignoring it for like cancer it grows more menacing under the surface!

SEE THE LIGHT TO AVOID A FIGHT

Thus it is very right to see the wild wickedness of people. Cruelty is subtle so catch it before it clips you. Become as skilled in its identification as knowing the stars. You must think: "she said that to get revenge." "He did that because he can't control me." Or "he wants me to adapt to what he wants." Whether you confront or not is not the issue---just knowing it's occurring stamps out denial and anger. You will soon be free of sorry conditions as depression lifts and your new light guides you free.

Cruelty hurts others but also the cruel one who is possessed by it. His first victim is himself as he despises truth and decency and anything else different from his own nature.   Many people aren't so nice and they love getting you into trouble. Can you not see this looking back? Stay awake--for a chief cause of sorrow is the inability to see through evil disguises. The worst part is the blind insisting they can see.

FREQUENT   FICKLENESS
Explosions of Suppression

Had you read their thoughts your past would have been different, right? Learn from that to avoid annoying involvements to which your center says "NO.". Notice for example how quickly people change their minds. They're friendly and helpful now but suddenly they're cold and evasive. Have you ever felt your protectors were your worst enemies? Don't be dismayed--these sad realizations symbolize growth into maturity. Let the tears flow! These are the floodgates opening you to the future and oceans of power. Down deep we all know the truth--it's just denial keeping us dull, dimmed, dumb, degraded--all delusions of the immature mind. You must face human nature to get the high prize of those set apart from the mass maize--the misjudgments of mistaken, masked identities. See them though it hurts. Then forgive--to take the throne as their leader.

You must dare to see through weakness posing as strength for staying in delusion is   scary, tedious and heartbreaking. Fooled once, it's their shame. Fooled twice it is yours. Growing up is giving up foolish infantile fantasies about phony "friends" and finding out those fallacious family fakes. The more familiar the pain caused by persecutors the deeper the knife—perhaps for your whole life. Think of the release about to occur--no more a sucker for the mockers. You want to be champion? Delete the fools and choose your folks. You must never rely on immature souls whose competitive strivings keep you down. As you learn to stand alone you will feel much safer with just truth and God as your teacher.

A cruel act is an explosion of suppressed energy. The pressure accumulates from having a pretense of being right when one is actually wrong.   So an inwardly wrong person is always under the pressure of this conflict which regularly erupts to cause pain and damage. But when truth takes inner hold he loses the pressure from pretense and thus also his cruelty. The phony ain't fine. He is gross and un-free: it's his envy you must flee. The greater your role shall be the better you'll feel as just "me".

LAW OF AFFINITY

The law of affinity says things of like tone vibrate together. Wrongness hates rightness and rightness parts from wrongness and the two can never relate--they walk completely different paths.   It helps to know that the faker of "right" is usually wrong. Getting hurt by wrong people signifies our denied wrong in ourselves which is attracted to another's inner weakness posing as strength. Yes the phony is blindly attracted to phoniness. You must be internally right to receive the safety of that rightness by avoiding the toxic system. This truth will guide you in all male-female relations as everything becomes smooth and pleasant. You'll instantly perceive someone's actual nature as meeting negativity becomes an instant warning against a disastrous involvement—for you've learned very well how romance/friendship with a cruelian is like living with a rattlesnake! No wrong man ever gets a chance to hurt a right woman as her rightnessness warns by instinct alone, and no wrong woman can ever deceive a righteous man!

FEARING THEIR ANGER

The most common fear is of another's anger. Knowing the nutty nasty nature of humans will lead you higher where you will say NO to your own fears. The prince will no longer tremble before the stubble. Only the weak wear wrath, yet you weep? You must now say "Cruelian I know you and will no longer shake under the tyranny of your rage." When you declare your independence and keep yourself safe these human storms will be of non-effect. If you can understand, you command. Shall I go on? By forcing you to give up on people your own inner journey will explode into ecstasy as you move into miracles. Detach from the outer: implode to the inner just by skipping dinner and avoiding the sinner.

The cruelian is a "vandal" who loves the thrill of hurting others. He is always playing games and repeating early templates to confirm self-greatness. Just when you think things are going good he falls into his bag: keeping you waiting, denying a normal request, forcing you into hardship and irritation. He digs driving you to desperation but he's weak so he's powerless. Just learn this type and you've won, then dare to disappoint demanders--never give what you don't want to give. Beware of expectations or being made to feel selfish and never be exploited just to satisfy them. Discern the valuable from the worthless--the egotistical cruelian has no value to you! As you wake up your responses to the harmful or unpleasant these instinctive soul-elevations will come from mind as well as habit. You'll see people differently and express it outwardly by refusing to "enter their den." No more your eyes glazed over with denial--now you're alert a rich squirt free of hurts and neurotic quirks (from being eclipsed by a shadow—not coming first).

EVIL HELPERS AND PROPS

The cruelian thinks for you--for a price. The most ineffectual are the most eager to help you. Refuse the charlatan's "two cents" and suddenly you'll think, act and avoid as you should. Your destiny depends on it. Involvement with wrong can distract or delete decades from God's plan for you. Avoid, then take control with perfect protection. And never forget the weak are a fake. Always ask: "what are you really like behind the mask? Since he knows he's false he'll either attack of flee. See that nice little lady? She's really a scorpion. Fakery is the cause of cruelty--so to escape hurt, see through masks.

CONQUISTADORS

The cruelian is compelled to win the debate, score the ego point, be a hero and demolish his fellows to feel good. He's a conquistador. Realize the danger here and instead of deflation think: "this could have been handled in a much higher way." Since a higher way exists, why settle for the lower? The conquering fool is just that--the low lured by like-lowness. He can never see the brighter higher world for a cruel man does not believe in himself. He tries to see his wrong as right but it's impossible--he wants his wicked ways to work but knows they won't. In conflict he can't believe in himself so why should you? If you do he'll hate you for your foolish flattery or fawning over a fake like him, so there is no winning in this situation. The fool tries to please the cruelian thinking he'll be loved but in so doing he becomes spiritually weak while declaring cruelty as worthy of worship! Why reward the ruinous, the recalcitrant, the rank? Some even fear rejecting this misery-maker. The solution is to realize you're not losing him but only your delusion that you need him! Detach, alight, see things right. Never fight just use spiritual might—transcend like a kite. It's your awareness alone that subdues those rising up against you, but your blind denial is the glue of gossiping groups.

ONE MONTH BIPOLAR (IN-OUT) DIET
Weeding Your Friendship Garden

They are either IN or they are OUT. Those who are IN you love, adore, cherish and reward. Those OUT you avoid, ignore, disconnect. Out of your circle they have no way in to hurt you again. You decide-- and when all is well with you there will be nothing wrong with your world. As it is, it's you sending invitations for disaster!

Practice IN and OUT for one month. You will feel more relief than you've ever known. Once someone is designated OUT your inner man realizes he's a foe or a faker and so attaches no significance or expectation to the contrary. Thus he is no longer hurt by unexpected slights or slighted expectations--there is no hurt nor salutation for the King salutes not the foe. Just stand upright and keep your head above the cruel crowd through aristocratic reserve. Be terse, laconic, sober. Give no account nor take thought for the OUTS and love to their death the INS. In becoming King or Queen the OUTS will never slight you again--they hate you anyway for placating, pandering to and pleading with their sick, silly and sadistic souls. Some men only love those who can see right through them. So if you want his love designate him OUT--only this brings the respect precursory to love.

TO BE KING AND QUEEN

Make people win your favor by growing up while never trying to win their favor again. Your new matrix of IN-OUT will form a new future as good as fame and fortune, for in so getting your world organized the relief from tension will open the floodgates of newfound energy— its like an ocean going through your veins. It's an easy way of asserting self in sweet silence, as silence says it ALL--they all know what they did anyway so there is nothing to say. Your silence is a siren suggesting they spurt up speedily or "so long, so-low, I'm going solo." Since all misjudgment is oppression (indicating wrong people) the IN-OUT matrix removes the block keeping you from success.

BRINGING UP THE BAD (PAST)
Labels and Fables

Cruelians are big on bringing up your (bad) past. Think ABM: Attack Bad Memories. When he hurts you this way just remember that (1) he seeks to weaken and confuse you to inflate self and (2) you aren't that same person years or seconds ago for the True Self is new every minute. Take a rattlesnake and call it a "kitten". It's still a rattlesnake and visa-versa. Ignore people's insults and self-flattering labels and just see realities. They call themselves "loving" to veil a viciously vindictive mind. It's the "humanitarian" groups which often hog and horde power and wealth. Stop believing in labels especially those put on popular people and petty past-times. See their inner realm--you cannot afford not to for the time is late so give up on the cruelian who always excuses brutality—thinking he's a right to attack, to rub your nose in your past or to betray a promise. When he justifies, he lies! Worse, his cruel crony counterparts support his hypocrisy while his very victims see him as a charming though rough "liberator".

SECRET WORLD

To detach, live in your own secret world. We can't change unpleasant people but we can unchain from them through a "secret world of safety." Never let them know how childish and ignorant they are. Keep your wisdom to yourself and your secret world is a happy world. It's so nice to live in the desert as I can turn from man, mass or mess to face the beautiful mountain vistas, the eternity represented there in pure sun and air. Suddenly I get caught up in the miraculous moment and all goes "strangely dim." Everyone's on probation here for in the desert wilderness no one can compete with eternity. This is the mistress we should always turn to when people problems persist. Go tell it on the mountain then the OUTS dissolve or die and the INS co-enjoy the eternal ease and evanescent ecstasy of living without obstruction (oppression). Your phony friends or flimsy family have contaminated your aura---and you can now de-contaminate by rising out of their reach to real regality. Turn to eternity when all such paltry petty people problems and politics is past.

POUNCER

There's more to say about the cruelian, who is a pouncer. He's always looking for an excuse to scream, attack and injure as his cold eyes resemble a wild animal waiting for his moment to pounce. He loves making you nervous about every word you say. The pain of persecution from cruelians dissolves when you understand it at this higher level: By seeing the incredible pressure between their true and false identity we can end the pain caused by troublemakers. They explode with (often "polite") cruelty as a bio-device to release the misused energy. They are helpless--seeing this will switch your state from fear to insight. Perception prevents pain but refusing to see what is going on allows the cruelian to confuse, cajole and cause you to cringe. Its like putting a blanket over your head--the blanket being his anxious face, resentful words and empty life which strikes fear like the desolation of hell. Putting you in constant fear is his invisible crime as his defeats become your worries. Let recurrent outbursts become a blessing, for visions spring from crises! Use terrible traumas and tantrums to reveal solutions while giving you the will to act on them. God doesn't want you to be mentally accosted and destroyed by evil--only seeing through empty (though glittering) social rewards brings joy so ask yourself: "do I want to be here with him (them)? Success comes with seeing through the world's false front and "fun"—it is foolishness.

HIGH CONQUERS LOW

They do wrong because they don't know right so when hurt always think "the higher conquers the lower." Unconsciously they act superior assuming the pecking order is right and you are wrong. Don't struggle to win--just let God's higher force act for you. It's society vs. God who is on your side and soon all will know it. Never expect compassion from a cruelian for he's always looking for revenge and destructive ego-thrills compensating low self-esteem. Stand in "high silence"--so high science can make his effect null and void. Since it's for want of attention that bullies behave brutally they crave to be fearfully noticed with screams or arguments—so your non-reaction is their confusion and defeat. Test cruelian's terror from being totally ignored: casually ignore, then carefully watch as the hurtful hero becomes a crybaby. Your denial of what he's really like only means one thing: the sly sadist succeeds in leading you to strife and sadness. Has this not occurred all through your past? You deny, you cry. You buy that lie, then to self-esteem—bye-bye.

SUPERIOR INSIGHT

Now you can see people in an entirely new way no matter their social image. The hard-hearted are miserable, the cruel are lost and the touchy have only pretensions of happiness. Vernon adds that the vicious or vile actually take their own pain as pleasure "preferring self-destructive attacks over a peaceful existence." It actually gives them a painful thrill. Don't forget the harder they fall (e.g. in love) the quicker they'll turn on you. When trust is lost, it's lost. Some sneaks are like snakes--they suddenly strike then slither away for good. They go UP at your expense then way down. Superior insight is the ability to see the reversals and ferocious flip-flops of people: friendly in private they suddenly switch when surrounded by "familiars". It's a case of OP-TRUTH: all men are two (opposite) people in one as there are two sides of the brain and two separate nervous systems. The private and social sides may be worlds apart. It's your denial of the two disparate sides that makes life so difficult, so to avoid disaster think: "it's a package deal" and then decide--wait and see as Jekyll becomes Hyde. You get their help, but soon you'll yelp. And thus it is keen patience preceding your triumph, not bitterness or wrath—just calmly taking note, then take a new boat.

NEW BAG OF TRICKS

The brutal man cries he's changed his ways, appeases with apologies then strikes again. When he cries he lies. Though a snake learns to kiss he's still a snake. Catch cunning cruelty by asking: is it ego or truth which causes his actions? Since truth doesn't deceive you know conceit caused the cruelty--and exposure makes it powerless. The cruel gang always demands you plan for their benefit so just casually ignore and plan your own right life in which they have no place. Take charge!

For those of you who don't know cruelians this may seem misanthropic and negative. You fortunates don't have an early template repeated through life, but even you will witness people-pain. Preventing its place provides a peaceful view. With a new mind you'll see the connection between your fear of someone and their behavior towards you. Your anxiety is a negative magnet to the hurt you believe the harsh can inflict, and just seeing this attracts a higher mind. Stay free of psychic violence by being an anger-detective of all hostility. Here's the clues: sudden silence, sly sarcasm, sullen stares and silly submission. Other common signs are forced frivolity and "coldly polite accusations." This knowledge allows your disconnection from emotional memories putting you so high they can no longer reach you.

STRIFE

Strife is a killer--a demon sent from hell to ruin every project or relation you have. It's name is malice, envy, jealousy, anger, resentment and bitterness. It's a spirit let into your life through sin--of act or association. Getting caught up in strife means we totally lose the anointing--the tangible power of God along with all our spiritual gifts (they're gone with the rifts). The cruelian wants to involve us in strife so we must do everything to stay free, for our very life. Most stress-based disease derives from strife—to the nervous system, organs, and tissues it's like a knife. Residual resentments cause disease--everything from asthma to warts. That's why we must understand cruelty lest one is riddled with resentments and filled with ferocity without knowing why. The cruelian is in conflict and you were the closest victim, period. Wisdom about this is your shield while denial or ignorance means you've no power to wield.

LAW OF AFFINITY

The cruelian demands you vibrate on his low life scale. He plays a cruel note hoping for a tense or angry response which will make him feel powerful. Just play your high notes. For if you react angrily you demonstrate his power of control while encouraging his villainy as he senses your anger as weakness. Never consent to his level for your anger makes your feel defeated. Only your true nature independent of him/her will give you peace.

Every cruelian is an actor teaching you how not to live. Understanding will release fear. Remember that "even while smiling a cruelian is lying while always denying." So ignore his words--your "spiritual suspicion" warns like a bell so just listen to that and stay away. But he's promising rewards or rescue? Don't believe it--when you finally see his ever-emptiness he can no longer deceive. Just as you refuse to submit to tyranny he'll get the message and intimidation will end. Then remember: it was you who asked for the company that ended in such grief, so search yourself for unseen invitations and stop sending them out!

ALL'S A FRAUD

This is the era of spin-doctors and plastic surgeons. As surface appearance is all that matters, true character is lost. Machiavelli said "it's not what things are but what they appear to be." Everything depends on perceptions as reality--first impressions and image is all that matters for most so just watch out. But you stay deep and discerning and develop character (who you are when no one sees) for the double-minded person is unstable in all his ways. True character will eventually win out and bombastic false appearances will eventually always fail as an overnight success takes a sudden downturn never to be heard from again. Lies, hype and spin have no longevity.   Now embark on the diet of freedom--from any and all distractions from your purpose. Walk and live in truth and you'll be in the right, the prevailing light.

P.S.

Well you've seen the light and temporarily you have no friends! Don't get discouraged for now you'll get to know God real good. God knows your future—and you're in training. Jealousy is the biggest reason for anger--it's a common Biblical concept. People made you feel small until now, for gifts bring rifts.   They've wanted power over you to compensate their own lowness in comparison: those without power in God turn to witchcraft. Wisdom of God is all the power you need while transcending your weird world. Let the scorners scoff at God--fools hate knowledge! The world's wisdom and God's are opposites so learn to savor sweet saintly solitude.

4

SOLITUDE

When Free of Chaos Isolation Brings Clarity,
Pleasure and Mental Stability

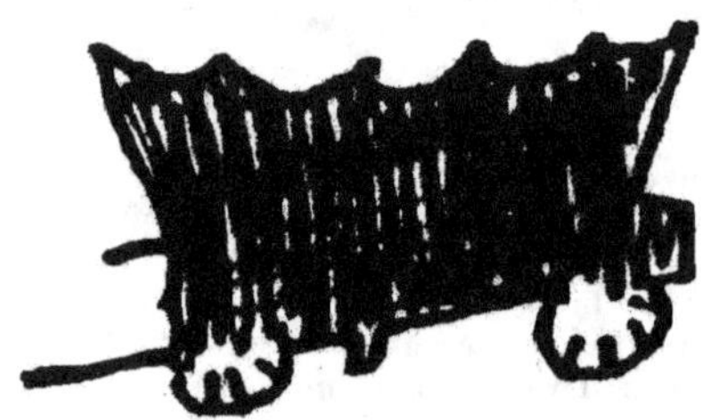

The power of the world is very strong as it beckons. The genius must learn to say "NO" and stand strong for his inner life, for it far outweighs the outer in importance to the self and the race. Then his grand intuition will be strong and redemptive endowing him with intellectual and artistic gifts, understanding and compassion.

There are two different ways of perceiving the world--through two different nervous systems (not one as old psychology assumes). The active mode is best for defending hunting, selecting and producing: it's a tunnel-vision which only focuses on the task at hand and screens out the rest which is most of reality—this is the basis of neurosis. The receptive mode is a diffuse, spiritual relaxation of this focused tension into wide-angled vision—this is healthy leisure and creativity.   Having let go of the extreme focus of the active mode the receptive mode takes over and miracles and insights can now be revealed through an inner journey. The cerebrotonic is someone who prefers this solitude with God and goes so deep that outer intrusion brings irritation and panic--he cannot abide casual drop-ins or chaos of society. If smart he learns to live a very formal lifestyle as he controls each minute of his day. He adapts to no one!

THE   INNER   JOURNEY

The cerebrotonic is so receptive he may have trouble distinguishing his own thoughts from the thoughts of others. When primitive he may act out their shadow, triggering the scapegoat syndrome. But if more evolved the mental static of social interaction so confuses it spurs a total retreat from social reality. This is a good and necessary phase in the evolution of genius as his smarts lead him to escape the severe undertow which gives no status to champions. If the aspirant doesn't understand this he may take on the projections of others and become withdrawn, submissive, anxious, disorganized, addicted. But if he learns to say NO to the world he can delete distractions and go deep instead. Then he'll be in touch with what the culture has repressed--the magical, mysterious, magnificent world of dreams from the depths of the collective unconscious. By his inner work he can retrieve these visions, return them to consciousness and reveal a cosmic unity alleviating the world's alienation. Look around--people have never been so alienated, depressed and addicted despite high-tech magic. This is because "where there is no vision the people perish."

BECOME   A   VISIONARY

As one embarks on an inner journey he begins to see the cosmos as a grand and beautiful design. But at just this wonderful point he misfits the world. If he can be free of remorse about this he becomes cheerful and excited at the inner and outer miracles occurring each day now that he can "see." Now that he's receptive rather than highly focused on action he can always be appreciative (quietly or ecstatically) of all of life's pleasures, and enjoy the creative insights from his leisures.

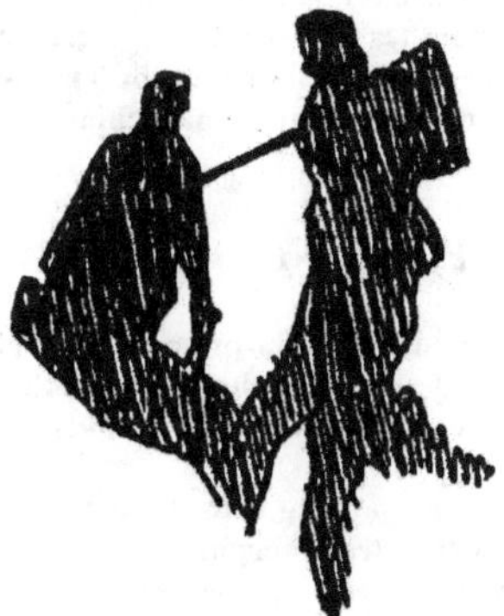

Just by going within one becomes a visionary. This makes it hard interacting with people less spiritually inclined for now there is a need to impart one's visions of awe and wonder— "pleasures evermore." Modern churches are often corrupted from the simplicity that is in Christ: to appreciate life as a little child--an awestruck curious happy kid secure in the arms of the Father.   The church charlatans want to complexify--add on--requirements for

CHAMPION GUIDES

Godliness rather than Jesus' way to simplify--eliminate all distractions and the superfluity of man's traditions narrowing all down to a simple loving relationship with God. These church legalists are "hard, sharp pressing and mean." Jesus disclaimed the empty traditions of the Pharisees and just said "take my yoke--it's gentle and easy to bear."

Without this divine relationship "religion" is the biggest attack on the soul, even more than the secular world. Someone has a sudden inspiring spiritual experience which leads him to innocently join a church. He then gives up his glorious freedom in God, facing instead a gray roadmap of legalism and requirements for salvation--so many he can never feel saved let alone happy. He didn't find a lamp to guide just a brick to carry. Where can the new believer go in generations which put good men down while gladly listening to fools and idiots? Where can he go when his own family may so resent and betray him--even selling him as a slave or handing him over to the enemy? To the inner world---the colorful infinite variety of rooms in his own inner castle. Once he does this God turns all-bad into all-good—for these very betrayals set in motion God's purposes for the misunderstood genius.

SOCIETY SHUNS THE INNER LIFE

The inner journey is very disconcerting to outsiders who have associated aloneness with thanatos, the death instinct. For women it is seen as particularly hideous. This became very evident when I left society to live in a small cabin in the desert wilderness. In complete solitude I turned inward and lived as simply as I could—even commuting by bicycle. People reacted with panic and disbelief as most would far prefer a crowded beach to a solitary island. The inner life just appears too self-involved to be healthy--we see adds for people with "social anxiety" as if the desire for solitude is a mental illness. This all comes from a Godless society and its social churches who see "being social" as synonymous with morality, goodness or Godliness. Little could they know that the True Self is universal (transcending family, race, culture, sex or historical era and all parochial ties) and thus the most important integrator of the world.

BODY TYPES AND TEMPERAMENTS

Cerebetonia is a temperament which prefers privacy and quiet order--and loathes chaos. Whether crowds or unannounced visitors both cause vexation, for this type only desires a vertical relationship with God not a horizontal one with his fellow man.

The three temperaments I describe go along with three body-types (soma types). The body of the cerebrotonic (private) is thin (ectomorphic), the opposite to the fat (endomorphic) which has a viscerotonic–extremely social--temperament. The mesomorph is muscular and his temperament is somatomic: he's into control, domination, striking power and defense. When there is any trouble all three react differently: The cerebrotonic desires privacy, the viscerotonic wants company and the somatomic focuses on action, defense, control and war.

In cultures where the muscular or fat predominate so does the social or defense temperaments. Cerebrotonics in solitude are often judged insane, but people have a right to their temperaments which are quite normal for them. Society hopes to re-educate them out of their reclusion to treat their "social anxiety." Treating them as socially deviant is a false philosophy for they don't hate people--they just love and seek the company of God. They love letting the mind spin to eternity while sitting in the collapsed moment where past and future unite. No "conversation" with an outer adaptor can compare with this rich luscious "fat" pithiness to each divine moment. As seeker and God unite the genius naturally unfolds to the unique self which God designed. This recluse just wants to reach his full potential before he dies--the completed blueprint design of the Creator for him and him alone—and cannot abide intrusion into this most important endeavor both for himself and the race.

Compared to the continuous revelations when alone in nature, man is a bore! Most people revel and enjoy the world's chaos from which the cerebrotonic retreats in haste. In this generation we see an aversion to order and purposeful disorder--to the cerebrotonic this dirty disorder is hell. He cannot abide the "slob" or loquacious talker who can't differentiate the trivial from the important and is steeped in banalities--current styles of "thought" or the "politically correct." The cerebrotonic adores the higher life evoked through clean order and thus he prefers to be alone.

In extreme cases the cerebrotonic is like a savant autistic. Autism is being in one's own world. It includes all IQ's from genius to retarded but the savants are brilliant (inspired--their work is automatic) though socially "dysfunctional". They have definite characteristics: they can't live with people nor can they be married, they prefer to live with animals and always in nature, and they react with long-term panic with unexpected arrivals. They have the inability to adapt to people--and a lack of desire to do so lest genius bog down in the dense.

It is the clash of the three temperaments that often ends in the demise or downfall of the unpopular cerebrotonic. He must be educated about people like himself vis-à-vis people like them. Then his power can develop as it is supposed to--magnificently as he makes the dent he is designed to make. If the inner journey may get lonely on the way to success there are six points to remember when readying for the comeback:

1. After a lifetime of wrong living, treachery and betrayal if it didn't kill you it only made you stronger. Just rest now--you must convalesce after all of this. Look forward, for God has a plan for you. Fear not.

2. For every great task a man is born. Your vision is true and real--it just takes character building to achieve it. Overcoming all obstructions through the Inner Journey is the path to the Great Work.

3. Expect your isolation to bring controversy. "A single woman is an untold story and a curiosity of interest." Particularly for females, isolation might become a silly or sorry stigma. You must know you're right and just do your work.

4. Have no more part of secular culture. The world will confuse you as the battle for the mind ensues between positive and negative, success and failure. Too-much mixture is our downfall! Stay steady on the course and allow no distractions. Just say "no."

5. Human greatness is known when it is *seen*. You've been transformed but still there is no progress. Realize that "they" must see you for the great inversion and then success to occur. Physical purity makes you Great.

6. Cast out all fears of "missing out." To rule the outer world you must go to the inner one. To stay partially hooked to the outer world will delay your success. You are missing nothing--dabbling in the outer means missing the Great Event on the inner. There is nothing to do, no one to see or "ask." Just arriving at that moment of the Great Divide when the outer reflects the inner and everything comes into order around you. It's all God's Timing.

SAVANTS AND ECCENTRICS

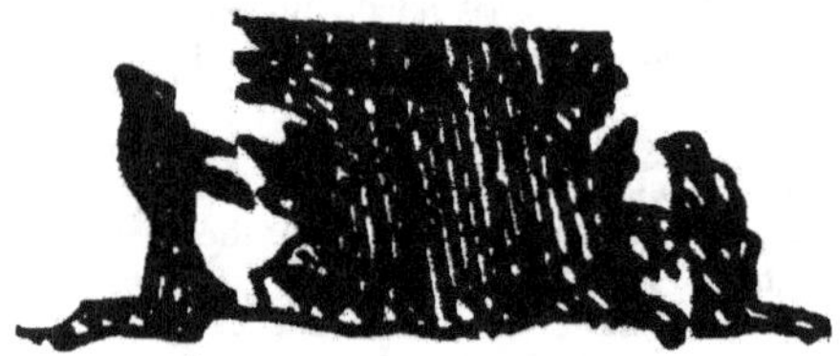

Chit-chat, logorrhea, trivialities, banalities, desire to be seen and belong--these are beneath the repertoire of the savant-autistic. The mature savant has learned to just sit there and smile until someone speaks with depth and meaning. Most conversation is superficial--nothing dare goes beyond "safe" boundaries without first checking the faces of the other "conversatants" for going too deep is nonverbally-punished in the interaction. For the Savant, listening to shallow conversation is a deadening chore compared to the kaleidoscope of meaning inside. This generation has 100 times the capacity to project words into print--yet the words are often so trivial, silly or copious. Yak-yak-yak: on they go trying to appear important to self and man, trying to be liked and get approval, appear interested and "loving"--playing to the gallery but never to God. To savant autistics like Einstein or Newton such chattering is noise pollution, static and a useless roadmap to nowhere.

"Eccentrics" describe these happy loners--the "strange hermits." The book Eccentrics shows that these types are healthier and happier than any other group whether married or single. Because they can't adapt they have far greater longevity for social adaptation entails so much stress it cuts life short. Though called "odd" they are the most intelligent, creative and healthy-minded of the race. They live alone because their "peculiarities" and sensitivities are hard to endure for those who have learned to tolerate (become desensitized to) the gross, vulgar, stupid and cruel. Psychologists estimate that only one in 10,000 is a true eccentric--like a landmark discovery, they are rare. They have been found to be nonconforming, creative, strongly motivated by curiosity, idealistic, obsessed about a hobby project or lifestyle, intelligent and opinionated.

Creativity is at the heart of eccentricity. Experimentation is the principal reason they continually challenge tradition--trying out new ways of doing things. They remain ever-childlike from when they constantly asked parents "why?" to the end of their life. Most become aware of their differences as children but for those who don't, tragedy awaits until they learn to insist on their own life. Eccentric children question not only educational methods but the philosophy behind what they're taught. It vexes an eccentric to adapt to anything or anyone--for it all seems silly if steeped in tradition or "group-correct" thinking.

Finding playground games boring and banal the young eccentrics escaped into books and other solitary pursuits. But instead of being miserable in their loneliness the eccentrics flourished. Freed from the need to conform that drives many people and wastes energy, they developed their own interests and agenda--and thus they were always happy. It never bothered them being seen as strange. History is full of eccentrics but most were male due to the historical bias against women. "Inconvenient" women were burned as witches or locked in asylums--unless wealthy enough to support their unique lifestyles.

Eccentrics develop in diverse backgrounds. Some are encouraged by parents while others torment the same with their defiant ways. In rigid fascistic systems they easily become the scapegoat never to get up again. In restrained religious homes they may rebel and turn against God only to find Him instantly when older and finally alone. Cerebrotonia--the love of solitude and going deep inside--is usually misunderstood by "outer psychologists" who have no understanding whatsoever of the inner journey. These "pros" are a dangerous breed indeed!

OUTER   PSYCHOLOGISTS

Since the outer psychologist is himself adapting to the social world which is sick, he has no sense of what it is like to go inward. He has a degree but in adapting to the social, becomes split. Dichotomized, he loses his psychology--then lives through his image as "psychologist" or "professional" while staying spiritually dim-lit. Living through the image, he must control the patient--make him adapt to the social world--to buttress and enforce his own failing and weak social reality. Cerebrotonia--a wonderful race-saving thing--is squashed under the big bug of social hebephrenia calling itself "professional." The same thing happens to the lone anorexic. As the others consensually validate themselves as superior they gang-up on the solitary anorexic, an easy target. They must scapegoat to confirm their false reality, for the social is not superior--it is usually a waste of time.

After years of solitude the eccentric becomes increasingly different from the social drumbeat. If weak this gap triggers gang-ups but if strong it is precursory to success--for those very persecuted differences will change the world soon. After years of such treatment the eccentric must now find peace--for he is coming closer to the truth while the others are farther from it.   After living in isolation just everyday conversation seems a hodgepodge of nonsense and meaningless hilarity. People really do think that social involvement is "Godly" and that the recluse is evil or sick for in the twentieth century people-worship has replaced God-worship.   Outer psychologists never question their premise but assume their own misinformed mal-adaptation is "right, good and proper".

GOING SOLO IS THE BULL'S EYE

Going solo is being right in the middle of God's will, and this is power. Solo hits the bull's eye every time! Letting others in to interfere with   carnal "advice" warps one's intentions and divides his power. At first it feels vulnerable to be alone, as if strength comes in numbers. Not so with God, for being alone is essential for completion and success of the Creative Act.

Look how they're all running out for entertainment. Yet one of the worst things about war is being taken out of your home--your power base, protection and reflection. People expect you to leave home lest you "miss out." Not so—going out means missing out on the private, mysterious, richly-powerful inner journey at home. Outer psychologists remind me of the Nazis who even forced their own people out of their homes. When I was a child my sister and I were sitting by a pool at a country club. I was enjoying the sun and the ambience. Suddenly she insisted I talk to the girl sitting nearby prompting me to be "social." Since I was in my own world I refused and she became incensed. That always stayed in my mind as it was so often repeated since. The world and the professional have no understanding of the inner life so we must up-level its status to evoke True Genius in the revitalization of culture.

The inner journey is so beautifully described by William James speaking of the saints in history. One said

"I was brought off from all outward things…to rely on the Lord alone. I forsook the priests the preachers, the most experienced people for I saw there was none among them who could speak to my condition--except Jesus Christ. I realized this only when all hopes for the others were gone and when I heard it my heart leaped for joy. The Lord showed me there was no one who could help me but He. I had no fellowship with people, priests, professors--I was afraid of all carnal talk, talkers and talking for I could see nothing but corruptions. If I had the King's diet, place and attendants all would have been as nothing for nothing gave me comfort but the Lord and his power. I saw how professors and priests were whole and at ease in the condition which was my misery, loving that which I would have been rid of. But the Lord gave me all my desires and took over every care--upon Him alone do I depend."

James shows how this "genuine firsthand religious experience" evolves: First the prophet appears as a "mere lonely madman" but if his doctrine is contagious it becomes a definite heresy. As it grows enough to triumph over persecution it becomes a popular orthodoxy. Though the faithful live on the original revelation the creative spring eventually runs dry to be replaced with dead dogma. The point is the religious experience lives itself out privately--it is personal. It comes in naked and lonely and it always drives the bearer into the wilderness and isolation:

"Having forsook all evil company I took leave of father and mother and all relations. For I durst not stay long in a place, being afraid both of professor and profane: lest being a tender young man I should be hurt by conversing much with either. For which reason I kept much as a stranger seeking heavenly wisdom and getting knowledge from the Lord."

After the new church becomes popular it stifles the spontaneous religious spirit while ignoring all new revelation. If a church member decides to stay home to ruminate, fast, study or go deep inside the parish will visit and chastise him for not attending church. Any sign of inwardness is then seen as "ungodly" while social attention at the pot luck dinners is "Godly."

The fact is that "men's minds are built in water-tight compartments. Religious after a fashion there are many other things inside besides religion and unholy entanglements and associations inevitable obtain." This means the churchgoer suffers a contradiction between what he says on Sunday and what he actually does or thinks. This is due to "religion's wicked practical partner": the spirit of corporate dominion which masks all contradiction through dogma and rigid church rules. Dogmatic dominion covers contradiction by laying down the law in a closed-in theoretic system. The result: an inborn hatred of the alien, eccentric, non-conforming one as an alien. Piety is the mask but the inner force is tribal instinct." Strong affections need a strong will. Lest they die as scapegoat-outcasts the savant must be strong enough to keep intruders at bay and maintain unabashed reclusion. Strong powers need a strong intellect which needs strong sympathies to keep life steady. It's the purely interior life that is the most likely to succeed. An overnight success can fall swiftly from fame and fortune. Your talents will take you places but only your character built on years of inner work will keep you there.

SAINTLY AUSTERITY

Austerity has great rewards. When the saints reached the point of no-people and all-God, love and family became interfering distractions from this all-encompassing power. This narrowing of focus is simultaneous with acute sensitivity, as suddenly everything is just too much and only the inner journey satisfies. Now the saint requires a simplified world to dwell in, as variety and confusion requires too much adaptation. His life is unified just as the "specter presented to the soul" is simplified. A mind extremely sensitive to inner discord will drop one relation after another for interfering with his absorption in spiritual things. Amusements go first, then conventional society, then business, then family duties until at last perfect privacy—sweet saintly seclusion. Lastly there is a subdivision of days into hours for specific acts like arising early to write, errands and housework, the daily meal, and contemplation. The lives of saints are a history of successive renunciations of complication, one form of contact with the outer life being dropped after another all to save the purity of the inner tone.

At this point silence is the rule so as not to sin or offend in social circles. If the life remains a social one at all, saints from all religions follow this rule. The zealot for purity feels clean and free only when "embosomed in monotony". The minuteness of uniformity is something inconceivable to a man of the world. Dress, phraseology, hours and habits are absolutely stereotyped and in some people this is incomparable mental rest and joy for the more uniform life's routine the more time to enjoy the day with God.

5

FALLEN HERO SYNDROME

*It's Always Tribalism vs. the Loner. If Strong he Becomes
Shaman but if Weak he is Dropped or Killed*

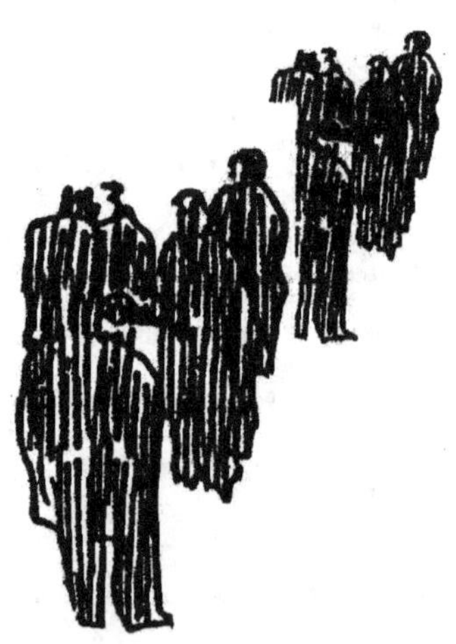

In purity he suddenly shoots to star success. In impurity he spirals down just as fast. Sin cannot be predicted--it will keep him longer than he planned, cost more than he thought and destroy all his dreams--shockingly and suddenly. It's not just the sin that brings him down--it's also other people as they get involved in his decline. Such is the process of the Fallen Hero Syndrome.

Our hero begins as pure raw talent voted the most likely to succeed. He has obvious and great potential—he is meant to rule and lead. He moves up to the plate but is too weak due to his sins which bring vacillation of mind and talent. First he's conducting the spirit, next he's refracting it into sensual pastimes that warp, dull and degrade. Having refused to stand up, stay strong and do his duty he falls at the hands of an angry jealous mob who tries to kill him. Because of his strong spirit there is no in-between--either he leads and gains their respect or he loses and brings their impulses to slay. For jealousy inevitably explodes against the great-going-down: "who did he think he was trying to rule us?"

Once he begins to slide down the down-spiral takes off and nothing can change its route. The consequences of sin are inherent in the sin itself--sin contains its own punishment. He's getting weaker and is shocked at his sudden decline, then the others chime in to seal his demise. It's just like chickens: once one is pecked they all gang up and peck to death. Again people and animals are much the same.   Man acts first then justifies through the frontal cortex second.   Such is the scapegoat system which surrounds alcoholism, anorexia and all other disorders: It's very hard to get up once you've been down. Only true champions--the overcomers--can pull themselves back up through the only answer: repentance. Then they must stand up and resist the undertow to fall back to the status quo. Repent, then act like nothing happened for it didn't--sins erased, no longer habit-encased. It was only the ongoing habit that made it real. When it is truly over, it never was! The fallen hero stays down only from cycles of sin and human systems.

TRUE GENIUS IS EVERYONE'S BIRTHRIGHT
Unleashed Through Repentance

We are born as unique seed potentials containing all of our potentials and peculiarities. This is our true genius, our blueprint-destiny, the easy-flowing talents that define us as an expressant of God. As easy and effortless as a bird singing, if we can just find this groove we have it made for life. But it's a mere dormant potential unleashed only through repentance. As such very few develop it, for in this generation they don't even realize they should repent.

REVELATION OR AUTONOMISM?

Beyond the scriptures unique instructions are revealed through revelation. But never trust revelation unless you're pure. When in sin there are "autonomisms"--up-rushes from the unconscious: twisted, uncontrollable thoughts and deeds. True genius is only from God and the dark sinful soul remains the bad act, the would-be genius, the mere potential, the "has-been-who-never-was." What is sin? Look at it this way: Einstein has proven it's all just energy. Sin is recycled energy in outworn channels--it is pure repetition. Quick-to-shoot and grasping carnal drives block energy and the "serpent" recoils tighter each time one gives in to the drive. Each time it becomes easier for the bad memory to trigger the craving to sin and we lose public and private power. But with repentance there is a spiraling release of this blocked energy up the spine and we are saved from the drudgery and misery of the sin-filled life. The biggest reward of repentance is unleashed forces--the blueprint potential at birth: our work. Never trust your revelations until then.

With repentance we experience a psychic opening: like splintering glass pure light shatters the darkness of sin. Oh happy days--one wonders why he waited so long to give up these useless burdens. The exhilaration of sudden energy unleashes our True Genius, an added reward beyond pure joy. With their conversion the saints were overnight successes: Having fruitlessly striven for decades their work now blossomed to the world with God and the angels bringing the Great and Marvelous Work to completion. It was as if the ex-sinner-now-saint was being carried downstream in spite of himself. So relieved is he that we can see how the greatest (and most grateful) saints were the worst sinners, for they had the most to be happy about!

BLINDNESS IS THE PROBLEM

To sin is to miss the mark--the blueprint destiny at birth. Worldly approval pales compared to this true success. These potentials--which God will surely further--are impossible while in sin. God wants us to express Him as He designed before our conception. What blocks this? Blindness is the problem. In times of mass sin and chaos prophets arise to tell the sinful masses what is obvious but hidden due to the blindness of sin. Because bondage is a bandage the wise and wealthy become fools "despicable, naked and blind." Because humans can learn to tolerate anything, prevalent sin is taken-for-granted as "normal." It is only rare strength--true nobility--that has independence from the masses and can take a moral stand. "Wide is the path to destruction but narrow is the gate to eternal life." The sinful man is too weak--he feels their strength in numbers and fears social disapproval should he take a moral stand.

CYCLES IN HISTORY

Many think the present moral breakdown has always been around--it's just "coming out of the closet" now. This view indicates blindness. The human race goes through cycles of moral degeneration/regeneration--ups and downs. In every case moral downs precede barbaric invasion--often from within. In the "ups" monogamy reigns, families stay together, people prosper, addictions are low and most are happy, self-disciplined and creative. There is order and simplicity--truth prevails. In the downs families disperse, men leave home, addictions are epidemic, prosperity dies and chaotic clutter (morbid accumulation) prevails. Through a process of gradual desensitization sin is increasingly tolerated (taken-for-granted-as-"normal") and the entire culture degenerates. Sin becomes a collective dark force, a mass amnesia called social hypnotism. The best example is 19th century England filled with unbelievable debauchery. Every generation has its favorite sins which become fashionable. At these times prophets function to tell the collective what is going on right before their very eyes but which they are too dense to see. The truth hurts (people love their sins) and the prophet is stoned ("they will hate you as they hated Me.").

CLUTTER AND CHAOS

Imagine a monastery with austere simplicity on the walls--a wonderful clean feeling of space and total order. Make your home a reflection of heaven--orderly clean simplicity--not hell:

dirty disorder and clutter. Imagine the truth of simplicity clearing the mind and releasing the exhilaration of real energy. Sinful man can't de-clutter--he's too afraid of losing it all.

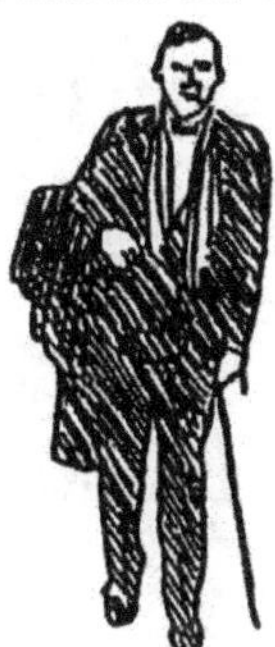

High boundaries = puritanical ORDER and then DISGUST with the junk all around. The saints have always sensed over-complexity and superfluity when in the presence of carnal man. For it is austere simplicity which characterizes the truth, the saint and the genius. The sinner is forever vacillating, covering his tracks, putting on a façade, dealing with guilt and remorse, justifying his actions, blaming others, planning how to get more, accumulating to compensate, trying to hold his life back from sliding downhill. His life is filled with compensations for sin but outer adornment (a loss of dignity) cannot cover evident darkness. He feels weak so fills the house with non-essentials, burdening himself with useless complexity like a dime-store or "tobacco road". The chaotic lifestyle is intolerable to the saint-genius who wants only the important to illuminate. To get to God's power we must have a prayerful life--leaving time, solitude and space for just that: concentration on the highest.

SPLIT-MIND: FLIP-FLOPS STING-SHOTS

The sinful man and his mind are dualistic--two people in one. Like the alcoholic, all habits create a Jekyll-and-Hyde temperament. There are two separate nervous systems: one opens up (in love) to the world and one shuts down (in fear turning to hate). Sin instantly switches to the latter shut down. When in sin there are no spiritual thoughts--only a dark cloud visible in the aura. One can't love, only find reasons to hate. Is their wrath amongst you? Then there is sin. Sin creates the fight-flight mechanism necessary for survival, so addictive perception is always shooting at shadows and looking for ways out.

Wild vacillations of mind--sudden "flip-flops"--indicate sin. The dual-minded has internal pressure from the conflict between who he is and who he says he is and this is temporarily resolved through explosions of anger--cruelty and "sting-shots": accusations and insinuations against those closest. These occur constantly but may be missed by others due to low self-esteem (sin blinds). Sin shows---in appearance, denseness, mistakes, broken relations and missed opportunities.   When in sin one feels (or misreads) the "cold shun" from everyone he meets.

CONCENTRIC CIRCLES AROUND SIN

Respect is innate for the True Leader of Men. Dignity is shown through purity and clear (innocent) vision. The true leader is loving yet takes a strong, unyielding moral stand. People get clear around such "warm steel" as the transformation of one changes the whole family system. In reverse, sin brings the contagion of madness as all are badly affected. Dark, disheartening vacillations are irritating and often dangerous though covered over by apologies and compensations. For all animals the mal-adaptation to hostile environments is exhaustion. All habits are pure repetition leading to this instability and fatigue as the mood swinging adds to the overwhelming complexity of the sinful life and adapting thereto.

FROM SIN TO SYN

The sinner is at a low vibration of reality in his own tunnel-vision. True reality is of God--it is cornucopia, a horn of plenty, a life of continuous miracles. With conversion we go from sin to synchronicity where everything fits like a jigsaw puzzle in the divine moment filled with cues, signs and symbols. As Jung said we should "watch for miracles like a cat watches a mouse-hole."   Each moment is a divine design--a blueprint-seed potential of the future. To sin in any moment means to warp the future, to seed for bad. If pure we go from weakly ordinary to powerfully unique--as we become universal and recognizable to all.   The Saints said much the same thing upon repentance from longtime sin: "I was riding on a wave of ecstasy and wondered why I had waited so long to give up this useless burden".

Here is the progression (degeneration and recovery) as we move from dense to clear: Born clear (unique), we are smashed and choked by the world--tamed to conform, our spirit is "broken."   Are you tamed to conform to the outright lies of those in control over you? Warning: herein lies the hotbed of denseness: attachments-through-denial. How to be happy: repent, break free of denial and enter a brand new life. You break free of denial by recognizing the difference between good and bad leaders (i.e. between clear vs. cluttered):

Clarity: High self-esteem, creativity, unique unfolding, receptivity, love bringing joy, pure awareness of the colorful now, growth, clear unbiased perception, spontaneity, cannot be controlled, aware of relationships.   Clutter: Low self-esteem, blocked energy, control, regression, tunnel-vision, fear bringing hate, past/future roadmaps and fears, repetition of mistakes, seeing the world through projections, rigidity, mind-controlled, hypnotized by relationships.

Many will forsake the saint and genius, having loved the present world. Can you still trust God, suffering and forsaken by friends and family? That's the trick—to win the test and be the best in whom all now invest.

6

ANOREXIC SYSTEMS

*Queen Ana: She was their Projection as
the Hate Group Ganged on her Past*

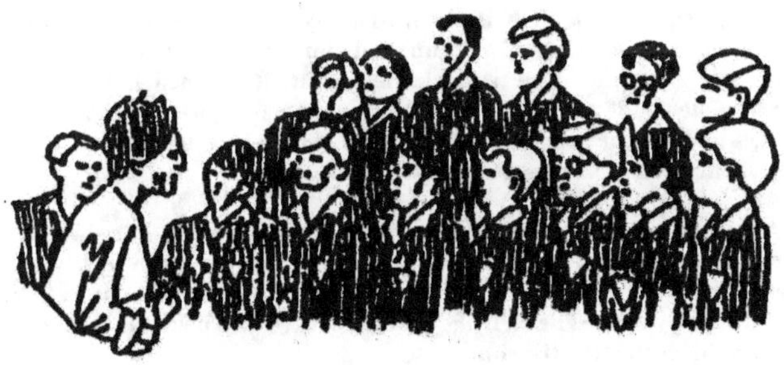

Author's Note: Extreme systems like that of the anorexic show what is happening to all systems to a degree. In all sick systems there is a group siding against one, secret alliances, redundancy of moral superiority, denial of change, no true leadership only group rule, and the making of the victim into a fool.

No one has power but that which comes from God. All we see around is false power--ego displays and tyranny. Ego and despotism is the compensation of false power which seeks to smash the meek which it reads as weak. This is the entire basis of anorexia psychosa--an ectomorph dominated and victimized simply by living in the   Land of the Big, Brutal and Brusque.   Ectomorphy goes with the cerebrotonic temperament which is totally misunderstood and rode roughshod over in the mesomorphic-endomorphic land of the opposite temperaments: social dominance and control.

At the basis of false power is social hypnotism: strength-in-numbers, also known as consensus--the "WE" vs. "ME." The misfit constantly collides with the prideful majority and is rarely accepted on her terms because like all genius hers lies in contrary instincts and deviant associations couched in austere simplicity. To the "dull normals" around her she seems inanely simple and mad, for she has the tragic ability to see through the contradictions which "everyone knows are true." Having things on her own terms is only her reward for having come through these group (tough-as-steel) resistances. She must forge enough strength and character to define her own way and go forth freely as Queen--for every day. But until then she must learn how to deal with those in power. Anorexia shows this conflict between the emerging self and the powers that be.

CREATIVITY IS THWARTED

She is born energetic and creative but meets a hard wall. As her creative self-expression is blocked it turns inward to creative self-destruction. Those with the dominant view are always jealous of God's power in true genius as they think they are Godly--because "everyone knows" the consensus is true reality. The power of group thinking or consensual reality is the herd.

The more energy she has at birth the more energy can be blocked and the more self-destructive she can become. Energy wells up ready for expression and meets an obstruction. If as a child your drawings drew ridicule that creativity turned inward, and thwarted creators can become "bad" or "mad". Since the energy must go somewhere it is misapplied to sin--recycled in outworn channels of bad habit. There it is, locked in a trap of despair. The most energetic become the worst when warped.

Picture it: As a child you are looking out the window pondering. You're in a beautiful state of meditation and contemplation. Suddenly someone attacks your reality and calls you "lazy." Your wonderful reverie is smashed and blocks inward. To adapt you curtail your own desires and act by rote. The striving to be is blocked and neurosis sets in to act out the false self while submerging the true one.

Energy is the same as spirit--it cannot be held down without severe and dire results. When this energy is finally released the result is self-expression--the talents of the True Self--and perfect success against overwhelming odds. If you feel exhausted then most likely someone is robbing you of energy, your most precious asset. People can't leave well enough alone-- though it ain't broke they still want to fix it! They want your attention--if it's elsewhere they rebel. You may meet someone and all is congenial. Then they discuss you with someone else, gossip degrades your image and they side against the Great as your new "friend" rejects and projects the mess back onto you. This is just human nature as it adapts in groups the fodder of soap operas: constant treachery in the pecking-order system.

I have seen the conflict between truth and social falsehood (or spirit and group tyranny) so often in psychologists who may know psychology but still want the approval of people. Despite their head knowledge they seek the approval of the herd. Dichotomized, they lose their psychology and become more blind than their patients. Having lost truth they work through the image instead, insisting on being called "Dr." to underscore their status in that system. Split, true power is gone while the image is staunchly maintained. Owned by the herd they persecute the lonely anorexic who jealously prefers privacy.

These "pros" are outer-adaptants caught up exclusively in an outer journey of negotiated meanings and current fads of thought. If the patient won't truckle to their promptings to become worldly, hostility emerges. We are now approaching a very dangerous situation with the authority figure in control and angrily wanting to make the other adapt. The "pro" must stay on top to confirm her image and while linking with the family she gains the tragic power to institutionalize the stubborn victim. This split between truth and image does not occur in a spiritual and creative society. So what can one do? Just self-educate and then insulate.

EARLY TRAUMA

We are all born whole and unique. So too the anorexic has a natural biological striving to "be" but meets an obstruction: a sudden searing shock called early trauma. Instantly all creative energies block and mobilize-for-emergency. The brain makes a template of the situation in a drive to correct it, and from that point on she repeats the same mistakes to correct the problem--but never can. That in a nutshell is neurosis: pure repetition acting in the present as if it is the past and never learning from mistakes. Not learning--the low "C" factor of all neurotics--is due to anxiety which we know prevents learning. The anorexic perpetually falls into the same old traps--of the group and her own.

For everything there is a season as normal human evolution takes place. But not so when a template is involved: things are stuck and stagnant--pure repetition. This stagnant redundancy is further frozen with sin---habits (like bulimia) to avoid anxiety from the template, the unfinished business of the past. To succeed one must be apt to receive. But the victim is not receptive to this whistle for she is drowning in the siren within from fear and self-doubt. The question is what comes first: the anorexogenic system (the system to which anorexia is a predictable reaction) or bulimia, incurring harsh punishments in the system? I hope to show it's a constant feedback for in any system there are no real victims or culprits, just a self-equlibrating system where all parts fit the whole in mutual reinforcement.

FASTING IS GOOD, BULIMIA IS BAD

Her sin and the system's template intermesh. They become one just as when drinking falls in with lower companions. Her answer is to release this wall of concrete and fly above like a bird---at all times looking down on the system and the world. She finds that fasting or just being thin allows her to transcend time and place and from this new vantage point (while still being stuck in a sexist and stultifying system) she becomes more powerful. The group can never be superior for in all eras its just consensus: "the extraordinary popular delusions and the madness of crowds." All through history the group was wrong, the individual right. Only in the fasting state can she partially prove this out. Eating, she is completely overcome.

The best example of early trauma, templates, systems and cycles of sin is the anorexogenic family system--the system surrounding anorexia.   Since anorexics are perfectionist-overachievers great success occurs when eliminating the influence of these systems and sin cycles. When purified it is now down to the attraction between like elements. Being an intrinsic overachiever and when mature becoming a perfect battleship, her success is inevitable. But let's review the early life of trauma to understand the fascinating evolution and example of the incredible strength it takes to overcome rigid systems. Remember most anorexics die.

ANOREXIA PSYCHOSA: EXTREME SYSTEMS

The young girl is not born with a "power drive" like most say. This "power drive" results from the thwarting of the naturally expansive biological striving to become and the feeling of lack of ability which compels constant improvement.   This thwarting comes from disconfirmation in a sexist system. "It's a girl"--only a mere girl. They may think she's cute but true confirmation of her possible budding significance as a potential VIP is absent. From this early frustration of the need to be. to feel and to have power, a "power drive" results to compensate for this deep gnawing sense of powerlessness coming from early frustration of expansion. Later acculturation only adds to the suffering, stricken sickened sense of self.
CONSTANT ENCROACHMENT

The anorexic constantly re-experiences the tyrannical constraints of relationships: imprisonment and frustration. It is vastly oversimplified to see this as "rejection of femininity" or "reversion to infancy." What she shows is a keen desire to become an autonomous adult. rejecting femininity which is the terror of just being a passive vessel. What she escapes is the negative part of social existence.   It is the stronger intellectual patients who seek emaciation and fasting as the magic key to greater power in society:

EMACIATION AS ESCAPE FROM
OR FASTING TO OVERCOME:

Non-acceptance
Ridicule
Exposure to lustful glances
Critical remarks
Aggression
Sexual advances

EMACIATION OR FASTING TO ACHIEVE:

Freedom
Beauty
Intelligence
Morality

Having endured the anorexogenic system which is so disconfirming the anorexic finds fasting a blissful state of well-being and overcoming. Body and spirit are now set free--the whole body-mind is agile and nimble. Material worries and irritations drop away. Her confines of reality are "YES" rather than "NO" as her horizons grow ever-wider. The spirit becomes sensitive, far-seeing and acute, the conscience quick and lively. She fasts to transcend the system burying her alive.

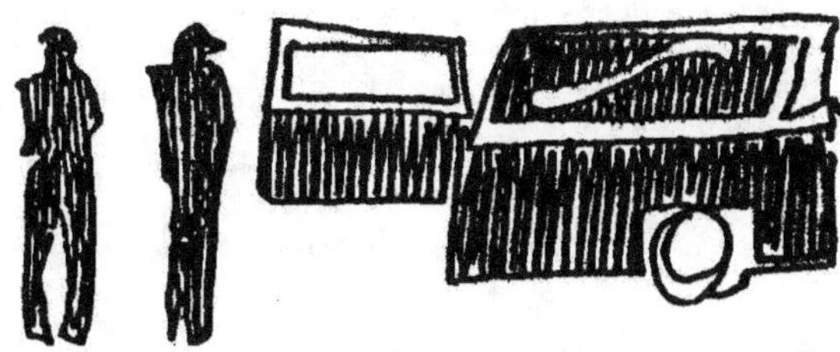

At this point she is hospitalized. Mere admission to the hospital, a rigid and regressive atmosphere causes grave emotional crises as nurses and doctors assume the role of severe parents. Her escape into "symptoms", her only means of preserving her autonomy from symbiotic and destructive relationships is blocked. When older the crystallized anorexic personality is considered incurable by the socialized pro who can't sympathize with her need for reclusive isolation. After a lifetime of encroachment, sweet solitude--precious privacy-- is all she wants. To understand this syndrome let's look at the anorexogenic family system, the most extreme example of all such systems.

CONSPIRATORIAL   CLIMATES

The home of the anorexic is a conspiratorial climate. All disorders are surrounded by sick systems but the anorexic system is the most severe. These systems have no true leadership: they just block communication through secret alliances shifting blame to the victim when any problems arise. To the anorexic they say: "I reject what you say and your definition of yourself (and myself) in this relationship." No matter what she says or does her image stays negative in the system. The family constantly stresses her "pathological" state of mind discounting all her messages while ignoring her improvements—and they do this by mutual agreement. This psychotic confusion between past and present is the rule of this system— despite present wellness she is seen through her sick past. As she refuses to be stuffed with food they'll say "she's reverted to a grave form of anorexic behavior" though the consequences are invisible. Let's look at the characteristics of families with these marked communication disorders to see how they maintain the victim's sickness.

LEADERSHIP

There is no real leadership--it's a group dynamic which leads. Here we see that the coalition (the group's siding against one) is the leadership. The group must maintain its identity (as having had the right in its superior position of mistreating the patient in the past) by maintaining the status quo. Thus everything the patient says is ignored or disconfirmed until she ends up thinking "the self is a fiction." Simultaneously no one leads because each feels a need to blame decisions on the others. About the illness they all say "there is nothing that can be done about it." The subject is not the patient--she is ignored--but the illness. The result is pathology in leadership for if nothing can be done there is no reason for anyone to take the reins and change with new circumstances. Thus the anorexogenic system is frozen like none other: a leaderless but rigid group mind. Here we see the principal of nonsummativity in systems theory: the whole is greater than the sum of its parts—it is the system which rules and the members are only mindless robots.

SECRET ALLIANCES
Cinderella Syndrome

The most serious problem is the system of alliances, the basis of a large number of secret rules that are never mentioned or hinted at but distort all patterns of behavior. Without true leadership there's just the group-mind goal of keeping her down and gossip makes the system run. Any mishap instantly shoots through the family grapevine as the group mind seeks to peg, punish, institutionalize. She is conspicuous against the ground of the pronounced sense of family, the collective identity with her excluded.

A very common system set-up with anorexics is the Cinderella Syndrome of two older sisters who are extremely hostile through envy, disgust and a sense of moral superiority. This is a triad which never changes: it's always the same two against one and the two always wins, the victim always loses. With their complete power and her powerlessness they can do whatever they want without fear of reprisal. She's long since been given "outlaw" status so the two sisters justify tough (cruel) love as "helping" the inferior and incompetent—she's a blank slate for all their deepest and meanest projections. As she seeks escape in God her life vastly improves only to be followed by their accusations of manipulation and deceit—for they disbelieve the invisible. This set-up is so unchanging that she either dies or pulls herself up in spite of it--gaining so much strength in doing so that she wins in all other areas as well. The result is world success, but it's all too-rare recovery from this mess.

ELDER ALLIANCES

The anorexic's symptoms appear after a change occurs in her link to the elders, her only protection from peers. Her siblings perceive her as having "special privileges" so as they grow in power and the parents recede the family equilibrium changes along with her presumed "privileges". As her siblings take control she is thrown down to the ground as her sickness takes on psychotic proportions. At this point self-starvation and bulimia become unconscious devices just to maintain sanity in this system--to carve out a self-nurturing niche and park there. But she is filled with shame--and if one feels shame people can always take more control.

GUT-WRENCHING ISOLATION

The patient begins and ends in isolation from the others in her family. Far from being allied with any one she is secretly detested by all. Her fatal loyalty to the older generation makes her a stranger and a resentment to her siblings. Friendships (her only allies) are never incorporated into the group but only criticized for being too intimate, assuming, gross, dull or morbid. Any new associate they will quickly dissuade against her--"how can you like her--don't you know what she is?" However if friends or mate turn against her and ally with the family they are instantly incorporated and even bribed for loyalty. This terrifying treachery seals her fate as she loses all faith in all human nature.   Insecure, she had desperate dependence on her mate and his turncoat status with the enemy chokes her soul. She spins down to psychoses after the ontologically fatal insight that the world was not what she thought it was. Losing all faith in man and herself, if she does not know God her self-destruction and death is immanent. She is squeezed out of the clan and feels so alone against the pronounced background of the rejecting family. She'd do well to read the Psalms: "I will not be afraid of ten thousand people who have set themselves against me". Even with recovery the clan puts on her a ban. For her own sanity she must realize she's the best and the anorexogenic system is the most extreme: She's recovered not only from a fatal illness but a conspiratorial hate-filled climate to which her disease was a reaction. But it's a feedback mechanism and a whole system. Her recovery can change that system since its pathology is the rigid (but leaderless) group mind that "things will never change"—so when she does (so drastically due to correct diet and fasting) it can shock them into the contagion of enlightenment.

BLAME-SHIFTING AND GROUP GOSSIP

The mothers and older females all see themselves as completely dedicated to the good of others. Their avowed generosity crushes all criticism of their constant encroachments preventing the victim's privacy or boundaries. Anyone who refuses to see the mother in this light is attacked. Even indiscrete promiscuous gossip is seen as worthy "to warn others about her." One anorexic said "My mother told even distant neighbors and acquaintances about my problems so everywhere I went I met similar hateful reactions." These constant self-righteous invasions are the very things driving the anorexic into cerebetonia (lifelong desire for privacy) and isolation. Due to lost boundaries and after such unrelenting harshness of her sisters everyone seems intrusive and invasive (see "She-Bully" in Ebook-6). Bulimia is a perverted attempt to establish these boundaries: by absorbing herself in food and cooking she is finally flourishing in her own self-nurturing reality which is normally "swallowed" by the family system. Food means "mother"--she is mothering herself since no one else will.

REDUNDANCY OF MORAL SUPERIORITY

In a system where her every word is rejected, rejecting food maintains this interactional style. Since he's the "professional" the therapist incorporates well into a system where all play morally superior. But in joining the superior group he is made impotent as he confirms their false view about the patient and her illness. He is paid to lie, to succumb to the tyranny of the   group. The whole communicational repertoire--rejection of messages, disconfirmation, invasion of boundaries, blame-shifting and secret alliances--are all highly repetitive patterns geared to keep things the same. The anorexic system--the system to which anorexia is the only appropriate reaction--is the most rigid and repetitive of all systems whether psychotic, depressant or alcoholic. There are so many interesting facts: e.g. with dual alcoholism in the parents 95% of daughters become bulimic. The eating function becomes disturbed in the context of constant arguments at meal time. No system shows more clearly how creative energy is blocked when the normal drive to become, to be and to be confirmed is lost. Energy blocked turns self-destructive. She fasts to become invisible since she already is in that system. Subconsciously her body seeks to reflect her missing selfhood. But the fast is also the only way she can feel good as a True Self.

HUMOR-HUMBLING

Humor becomes the system's defense mechanism: intelligent, witty exchanges and funny faces condescend towards the patient. These cruel evasions are performed so subtly and with such "good will" they escape detection, becoming a secret weapon to confuse and degrade her further. Humor can be very destructive along with other devices to maintain the system. The alert therapist should say "how can you stand these people who degrade you constantly?" But the outer psychologist who only wants to join the powers that be--and pay--says "why are you so bad or mad? Why can't you just eat right? Why can't you have congenial relations with your family?"

WEAK FATHERS AND THERAPISTS

If the therapist could be the substitute father the generation gap could open and the daughter could finally start living her own life. But kept in her maligned position, even far-off separations keep her obsessed with her oppressors in her thoughts, jealousies, resentments and transferences. She will see the same system played out with new people with her one-down. Her only solution is to embark on an absorbing inner journey which she already desires with all her soul. But due to low self-esteem, fear of being alone, supposed need for protection or "advice" or a need to feel confirmed she gets involved, stays down, feels invaded and often reacts with the same old devices of bulimia or starving. She must face and resolve the old system and her place in it, and the greatest possible outcome could be a mature lady in new town or family.

The best therapist would become an intelligent effectual father for the patient. Her own "ineffectual father" was the product of the same system--the co-op between the other members. Humiliation of the father was required to avoid changes, for a strong father requests change or adaptation to new needs but a group-controlled male tows the line--only to eventually be written off as his role is given to a son or son-in-law. This changing of the guard is pure disaster on the already invaded and despicably mistreated anorexic. The sons-in-law have had it with her and now that they rule their aim is to fix her for good.

EXPOSING ALLIANCES

To better combat perverse triangles the goal of therapy must be to expose them. These are secret never-acknowledged coalitions against one. Whenever the behavior of two betrays their secret compact the treachery is instantly washed over by meta-communication. For example one older sister gossips to the other about the victim who can always tell when they've talked as the first sister becomes mean (calling it "tough love"). If the victim confronts the pattern she is called "paranoid." This is the main pathology of the sick system: the coalition first, and the simultaneous denial of it, second.

A "coalition" is an unchanging joint action against a third person, in contrast to a shifting alliance in which two out of three people make common cause. Such dualities as good-bad, positive-negative and sick-well have no place in this cybernetic model of homeostatic systems. There are no "causes" just here and now the entire family collaborates to maintain the status quo (of two against one) and any accusation just hardens their self-defense (putting her down). They treat the victim's symptoms as "badness" leading to instant disqualification for respected membership in their morally superior family. This group hate changes the course of the disease from "nervosa" to "psychosa" as she takes on the sinister outcast archetype of the shadow–projections of others and her symptoms magnify. The feedback (mutual reinforcement) in the cybernetic system is evident.

What characterizes the family as system are the transactional patterns repeated with high frequency. These redundancies become rules maintaining rigid stability and the outcome are symptoms. Redundancy is most extreme in this system and thus the victim feels there is no hope--things will never be any different. She is literally made by these system etchings in her brain--she is programmed beyond her control. She becomes hypersensitive to people siding against her--she feels it and she creates it from the system template (her script). It becomes impossible to trust female friends. She wants to get out, to get well but is strapped in her chair while simultaneously being "hit" by what feels like outside forces demanding she binge, starve, seclude, go moot and suffer. Later the inability to trust defines her Queenship for now she can only rule and never mingle. To not rule means the Queen is lost--so she becomes hypersensitive to even minute changes in people's behavior--a characteristic of the millionairess.

BULIMIA: STARVED FOR IDENTITY

What these redundancies do is not "make her eat" so much as starve her identity—because the family refuses to confirm her. The meaner they get the more compulsive, unconscious and essential her eating device to keep some sense of self. Starving--becoming invisible-- makes things congruent with her missing self-esteem. She constantly makes new resolutions to act right, only to relapse into the same unconscious state. Bulimia or starving simply seems to make things better. And shame and embarrassment aside, it has long since dropped into the unconscious as just something she must do. But since bulimia causes more disorder in the system and her perception, she only gets worse and the system becomes more condemning, caustic, controlling and contemptible.

There are many who would judge the bulimic anorexic. To those judges I would ask--have you ever been in total anxiety all the time amidst a hostile environment--your own family who hates you? This is an environment in which you are ever-condemned without trial and it's always the same prejudiced jury. It's a system in which one is ever-trapped and -tricked and in which all positive changes are re-defined as negative. When evolved she will fast at her enemies never "eat at them" but in the weak and sickly stage through the reptilian brain she slides back into whatever works, the only "slot" there is. With anxiety or anger the brain auto-regresses into previously successful strategies all the while "food" means mother—she is seeking nurturance in the midst of hostility. There is no thought to such regression--its an automatic response to fear and her impossibly painful plight by slipping back into the behavior that "works". The anorexic is in the "burning building syndrome"—she feels there is no escape yet seeks it everywhere.

REDUNDANCY AND FAMILY RULES

The anorexic is blamed for all that goes wrong--everything is due to her illness. But a family is a self-governing system based on rules established through a series of trials and errors. All members are elements in a circuit in which no one element can have unilateral control over the rest. The behavior of one member is not the cause but rather the effect of their behavior. Family systems theory is the study of fixed behavior responses and their repercussions--- symptoms. But the whole system thinks the patient because of her symptoms wields power over the rest rendering them helpless, never thinking their own interactions may be causing her noxious behavior. What came first, hatred or habit?

This is a common error of Western culture and psychiatry: the idea of "self" transcending the system and hence being in control of that system (blame). And thus their reducing the victim to impotence is just the due and right response. Their tight and hostile alliance against her is condign punishment, and they can't see it any other way. Any attempt on her part to rise up is squashed, violently opposed and re-labeled. They must maintain the scapegoat lest they face their own part in the system.

Over-protectiveness, encroachment and prevention of autonomy would irritate any alert therapist who would also see how those in power dispense punishments, prohibitions or occasional presents to make their presence felt. Mixed signals from all the pretense abound so the victim mistrusts her own feelings. For example the older sister backed by the mother is envious of the patient's good looks and treats her with a mixture of concerned affection and great cruelty. This behavior sears deep into the anorexic's sensitive system--if her sisters seem spiteful and nasty it is because she deserves it! Binging and starving is all that lets her know she exists, that she can still feel, even occasionally enjoy.

RIGID HOMEOSTASIS BRINGS SYMPTOMS

The more intense the cold war waged by secret coalitions, the more secret. These pathological systems are governed by secret rules that shun the light of day and bind the family together with pathological ties that depend on the victim's one-down state. Her "symptoms" develop in systems threatening her demise for they act as submission rites to ward off aggression. The system gives her no choice but to escape and take refuge in her symptoms, for she has no avenue to creatively self-express--only to self-destruct.

In systems theory we shift the focus from the individual to the wider relationship. Here we see pure redundancy: anorexia is monotonous repetition as each member rejects her messages. The illness is always shrewdly presented in the same old moralistic and sacrificial tone ("symmetry through sacrificial escalation"). Without leadership there are only alliances against her, combined with blame-shifting. As time passes these patterns extend from the nuclear to the extended family (the sister's children are trained to hate her too) and any new acquaintances of the patient to whom the members "tell all" to dissipate their admiration. The victim learns to expect this and even in later years will never introduce any new contact to her family.

FAMILY VS. SELF

The collective sense of the family is so pronounced with her excluded that the lonely anorexic is increasingly pushed into the background. The family tends to stick together like a brood of ducklings. The grandmothers can play a major role in the family disorder and the father is so unsure of himself and afraid of independent women he married someone with many shortcomings. However intelligence, adaptability, culture, imagination and interests appeals to the father so he admires the over-achieving daughter but hides it when mother is around who becomes hostile and envious. This engenders more mixed signals and interlocking jealousy patterns. Female competition can be very cruel in this world. (See Jung's work The Three Sisters to see the deep and dangerous archetypes evoked.) Usually it ends in two against one and this constellation never changes. The victim never wins and gets used to always losing. But overcoming this turgid template can be done and the strength garnished to do so could make her a world leader in her field.

ACHIEVERS MEET SEXISM THROUGH FOOD

Sexism is a suffocating obstruction to achieving females as the energy turns inward. Perhaps they would have "chosen" alcoholism or drugs as their "sin of choice" but the loss of control, sure institutionalization or further degradation by family would have been intolerable to these types. Anorexia and bulimia are the only ways to recycle their enormous energy, ingather their forces, create their own reality, use their own time in their own way and still stay relatively in control of the situation. Anorexia is usually a feminine illness from well-to-do families. Why? Because these families often ensure smooth-running solidarity and harmony through authoritarian set-ups and the subordination of woman.

ENANTIODROMIA:
The Bottom to the Top, the Top to the Bottom

Having absolutely no control of the sexist system the anorexic drives this energy inward to absolute control of her own world--herself. If she can learn to turn lemons into lemon-aid and overcome this greatest obstacle--the stubborn system keeping her down--she builds a perfect battleship for war and the power to manage a huge world corporation. So great is her energy that when held down and turned inward she is the most self-destructive of all (bankruptcy, binges, brawls), but garnished and turned outward to good her self-improvement reaches monolithic levels. If she can learn to harness, tame and redirect this enormous energy she can greatly benefit the world of other persecuted pansies priming to push-up to powerful predominance. When she transcends all disorder (beyond mere eating patterns) and attains immaculate order in all areas instead, all that energy goes outward to world success. For those survivors the sky's the limit as the held-down energy bursts forth and catapults them up to greatest influence.

Like all systems the family tends towards homeostasis. But no living system can survive unless free to evolve to change when conditions change. A system dies if it has such rigid homeostasis that even the slightest positive feedback like her transformation is ignored. It will come back to haunt them as enantiodromia occurs: as the worst becomes the best. This inversion of systems means one goes up and the other(s) go down for nothing stays the same. When that whole homeostasis depended on her illness and she is now well and thriving something has to break. Throughout history the family was a homeostatic barrier against social change and the most rapid changes are seen today. Objections are eliminated in these systems by eradicating--making impotent--those who object!

ANOREXIA IS A SOCIAL ILLNESS

"A man's foes shall be they of his own household." Jesus also said that "he that loveth father and mother more than me is not worthy of me." Of particular import "a prophet is never known in his (her) own home or town." So true. For nothing the anorexic does can ever change the image--the leaderless group-mind simply redefines the new situation to suit the template with her one-down. Anorexic families are the most stubbornly resistant to change, causing a crises in a system from which there is no escape but to recycle energy inward through symptoms: homeostasis. Then her magnified symptoms compel the others to join forces to deal with her illness--as hand joins in hand they are more solid than peas in a pod. All group photographs exclude her, as do their parties. Gossip is the only way she is included. Otherwise when she walks in the room all turn aside.

Could there be any doubt that anorexia is a social illness, particularly since it is specifically bound up with the extreme system described? Yet hospitalization--although it removes her from the family--rarely brings permanent relief and generally causes deterioration of her state as it is just as bound up by hierarchies, demands and domination, sexism, deceitful alliances with family and disconfirmation of her. Any objections she may have to hospital food or any desire she may have to be fruit-fat-fastarian--the cure for bulimia, food addiction or failure to thrive--will likely be met with mockery and rejection.   It is all just "another facet" of her illness. They already know how her intelligence can justify anything with science research.

When all have turned their back on you and you still trust God while forsaken and suffering, the reward is world success and nothing less.

7

THE LOGIC OF ANOREXIA

Staying Free of Tyranny and High
in the Head: This is Mature Ana

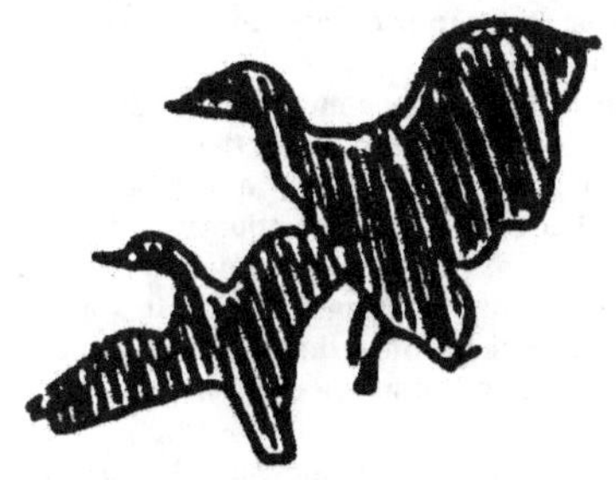

Author's Note: Fasting is good, and bulimia is bad. But if there is no bulimia I believe Anorexia Psychosa to be a most misunderstood disease, as some of the characteristics labeled "sick" are actually healthy or at least appropriate reactions to the system and predicament she is in. In this section I will illustrate this point and up-level the status of the much-maligned and lonely anorexic: full and food fears, isolation, insulation, cerebrotonia, ectomorphy, food discipline, order and routine, fasting used as a device to overcome, black sheep separation, aversions of lustful advances and aggression combined with eventual celibacy, separation from female culture, and her perception of many as frogs and toads (to the refined anorexic they seem carnal, absurd, obscene and vulgar).

INTRO TO SOCIETY AND GROUPS

The issue of anorexia relates to much larger issues about society and groups: systems theory, how people act in groups, how females are expected to conform, the implications of sexism in family-groups-church, what its like to be an ectomorph in a endomorphic-mesomorphic world, the signs and reactions of healthy individuals to domination, the acculturation process and how people take it for granted as mundane reality, what they do to outsiders or those who think differently, how female culture treats unique women (i.e. those who refuse to conform to the banal--those fashionable current "truths" which are simply fads of thought) and what it means to be politically-correct and what happens to those who are not. I say anorexia is the reaction of a hypersensitive who is aware of all of the hurtful nuances of humans in systems and that the characteristics below are just appropriate adaptation to that set-up. I contend that the anorexic doesn't recover--become a mature lady--until she acquires the Diet of Freedom: insulation into her own stream.

FULL PHOBIA

It is very inefficient to be full--all the energy is dragged down to the gut out of the head. As a birdlike engine, to the anorexic this can be a terrible "drag." East Indians laugh at how Americans are always eating and thus bringing energy down to the gut. It makes no sense, since keeping that energy high is where you get the genius, the inspiration, the brilliance as the spirit of God comes through, as well as the overcoming power over herd resistances to strength. Fasting is a matter of synaptic clarity--for pure conductivity to the source.

What becomes addicting is using food as a means of handling low self-esteem: eating when one feels "put down". The energy is taken out of the head to avoid the conflict between the real (how we see ourselves) and the social (how others see us) image. Eating is avoidance and thus becomes very addicting: As her situation with family and world degrades, her eating disorder gets worse since its function is a coping device. She binges so her self-esteem will be tolerable but when full or digesting she loses this power and purges to regain it. Fasting soon solves the self-esteem problem through a much more transcendent, happy view of life. The anorexic knows this and comes to use fasting to stay "on top" of things.

She knows the pure power of a clear brain, an elongated head, a beautiful face drawn taut from the fasting process, the sense of accomplishment that brings the necessary boldness to effect others, the spiritual elevation, clarity and inspiration--all from fasting. Fasting is not a sickness. Which group is sick--the eaters to avoid and stultify or the fasters to see and create? This culture is not into fasting—it is Dionysian, not introspective--so those who go inside are labeled "sick" so the others can maintain their delusion that "they need to eat." The anorexic has fasting consciousness--the others tend towards swine consciousness.

FOOD PHOBIA

The anorexic sees the relation between food and fat. Being birdlike she feels the effects of food far more than her heftier peers. They can eat anything and feel little difference while everything she eats seems to bring fatigue (energy down from the head) or that hated huskiness. She begins to feel that "all food is poison." At first she rejects all food but fruit, which seems pure. But fruit creates cravings and mood swings leading to binges--and great suffering/reverberation from her network like threats of institutionalization. The wise woman won't stand for that and ends up on a diet of fruit and fat which creates stability and suppresses appetite for long periods of fasting while still maintaining "normal" slimness—the recovered bulimic need never be seen eating again.

She's astute--food phobia is rational. Once one finds the problem it is wise to avoid it.   If she was bulimic she likely gave herself hyperinsulinism and suppressed immunity so as she matures beyond bulimia she may avoid sugars and starches to keep insulin down to eliminate mood swings, constriction, water retention, puffiness, hunger and craving, depression or fatigue. She seeks health and wealth through food restriction for it can never be gained through undisciplined eating. Food phobia is good, true and very wise. It's the difference between a great day and a damned day, so efficiency is not a disease!

ISOLATION

Its hardly a cerebrotonic culture--few embark on an inner journey. As the culture gets more superficial and shallow it also gets more carnal and vulgar--there is a wider gulf between the inner-driven anorexic and the fattening culture at "large." It is disconcerting being a tiny hypersensitive amidst the bigger and grosser who all seem to be dominating her life and telling her what to do. As a cerebetomic she hates domination--as the mesomorph's control and the endomorphs gossip, she feels squashed. Naturally she seeks isolation and delves into her own reality for even when they fail to find a flaw they forever pull the age card. There's no winning in crowds or clans when envy's all around.

The anorexic is constantly feeling the tyrannical constraints of relationships. As she matures she learns how to manage this disposition for a pain-free life. The issue is remaining invulnerable, achieved by being inaccessible and distant. The control devices that others see as normal she experiences as suffocating and cruel. As the social culture cajoles her to go out and do more, her solitude becomes ever more desired, inspiring and peaceful. She feels set apart—sanctified, even holy--though persecuted and despised. It is solitude that develops intuition and if maintained despite all resistances (the conspiracy against privacy) she will win every time. She is following the steps of history's spiritual giants spending years in the desert wilderness. Her true friends help her to glory in solitude and grow in intuition not "correct the condition" of "social anxiety personality disorder". How many genius cerebs have died through suicide or drugs due to this misdiagnosis we will never know.

INSULATION

For the hypersensitive, to insulate from chaos is enlightenment--a safety valve, a survival skill, a protection of one's own reality. If self-defense and assertion creates problems (as in a big family) insulation is the only self-defense. Her emotions are magnified in their presence as she takes the misfit status, for on every nonverbal level she is disqualified and knows it. It hurts being psychically attacked by their deep feelings of moral righteousness at her refusal to conform which is seen as "sin".

As the anorexic matures (and having been alone longer) she is surely marching to a different drummer. That is good--for she's a walking potentate of something big and so needs more holy separation and insulation from those elements advising her to join, co-mingle, socialize. It's really hard adapting to all those lies! Any joining would only restrict what is brewing under the surface, if allowed to develop on its own accord. The mature anorexic has had it with groups siding against, mocking or stigmatizing her differences.

CEREBROTONIA

The unique cannot conform to groups without cutting off parts of self. It hurts to tolerate stigma status, so being alone is bliss. The conspicuous are caustically and constantly misjudged in social cultures, so the recovered anorexic must insist on privacy--for the human herd is tireless in its malignant scapegoating and gossiping. When the mature anorexic learns to expect it she finally holds her head up high above the problem, for to not overcome the human element is to die--this is one illness only maturity can overcome. If she doesn't die she becomes the best in which all now invest. She shapes up by overcoming the herd's tendency to think like all one mind, by becoming a majority of one. Such insulation is one of the major factors in maturity: most people cannot sustain it as they run to others for confirmation. A famous female may be hated, but despite the hostile multitudes if she's found the True Self she can lead through aristocratic reserve: She maintains an inner circle of confidants and a poised, noncommittal and distant though cordial outer circle, and through this comportment she finally experiences true abundance.

The birdlike engine--the ectomorph--is just naturally cerebrotonic, desiring solitude when the "bigs" desire company. She has a vertical relation with God while the others relate horizontally to man. It seems a continuous petty sorority party with her excluded: She senses chaos and disorder of the modern world where children lack discipline and as it grits her nerves she either worsens or isolates into golden productivity.

ECTOMORPHY

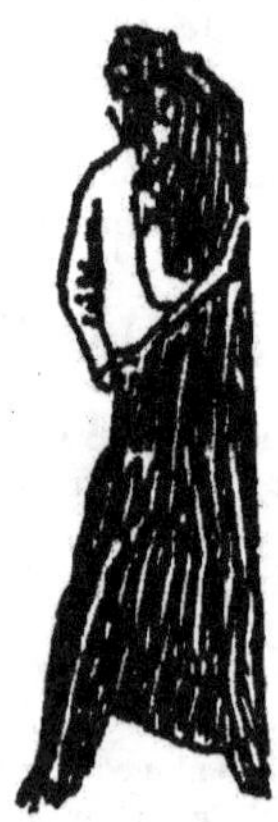

The thin ectomorph has far more surface-to-mass area with the lymph and nervous systems predominant. She is "wearing" her nerves and becomes whatever effects her as the social situation becomes acute and hurtful.   Being so tiny and easily ticked-off, any added weight becomes an intolerable burden so the immature anorexic becomes unstable, uncertain, unconfident, touchy. She dreams of future prosperity to transcend weighty systems bogging her down just when she feels up. She feels this ecstasy when alone with just God and her own identity--so reclusion becomes a must, as important as protein in keeping her structured and sane. With her, less is more and might does not make right. The ectomorph must learn the principals of non-reaction: let solitude and silence fight all battles.

FOOD DISCIPLINE

The anorexic is labeled "perfectionist-overachiever" as in this era champions are denigrated and victims have status. She demands discipline in all things especially food since weight irritates a touchy system. Most dieters get rule-sloppy, and the "rulish" are seen as neurotic. Without rigid food discipline one never experiences the great rewards of doing so, yet to them slipshod lazy discipline seems "righteous". Is it really wise to eat anything without fear of the consequences? Only in a lax society where children hate discipline and chaos reigns. To soar to the heights you must be rigidly concerned with food combining, sources of food, insulin elevation and periods of fasting. Yet to be this way she's called "orthoexic" with very hostile reactions to her fasting. It doesn't matter bliss or beauty--to the slovenly socials, discipline is "sick."

ORDER AND ROUTINE

Cerebrotonia is fear of chaos. It is hardly neurotic to see that chaos is hell and dirty disorder or that order and discipline brings happiness. But in the new age of lax-seen-as-freedom it seems neurotic and the anorexic soon learns to hide her rigid routines. If living with others less inclined she may be sabotaged or deliberately messed up to "help her to relax." For the structured anorexic, living with others can be a harrowing experience and will surely end in relieved isolation. Her high goals are only possible when free to be a "strict methodist" of military-like routine and order and this means being alone. Going deep with God means saying no to many surface things--then it's her soul which sings.

FASTING AS A DEVICE

All she wants is what everyone wants: love, acceptance and space, and in a social culture this is only possible through solitude. If that's not possible she's learned that fasting works for beauty, self-confidence, wit and transcendence; and that eating and digestion only brings the energy down--a tremendous loss. Fasting has been used in all religions since the beginning of time--it's the universal device to get to God's power and is always followed by reward--like resolution to a problem, overcoming an enemy, success, health. In this Dionysian generation of anything-goes you're-not-going-to-tell-me-what-to-do rebellion against all authority including legitimate rules or decisions --fasting is definitely a lost art. I once joined an Atkins discussion list on the internet. They were all for eating meat, as much as you want and as many times a day as you want, yet when I mentioned combining it with long periods of no-hunger fasting they angrily threw me off the list. It was extremely telling, for the joys of fasting ecstasy and bliss is lost in this me-now generation of nothing deeper than the taste-trip. The anorexic knows the joys, extreme efficiency and sacred spirituality of fasting and this is her grace and blessing--not her disease.

BLACK SHEEP SEPARATION

Any hypersensitive slowly or quickly edges into outlaw or black sheep status from the group as he reacts adversely to what others see as "normal." This is difference enough but adding those of eating habits--like food restrictions or fasting--completely sequesters one from the group. Whether in family neighborhood or office the ana easily evolves to the conspicuous or cat's paw. Like any stigmatized position every act becomes caricatured through misjudgments and gossip--such is the plight of independents acting to truth not conformity, to whom all groups side against. If she knows about insulin and refuses the bread she becomes a sore thumb in circles valuing the "norm". All groups and female culture at large act the same way. If you refuse to conform they mimic, mock, deride, hate and slander. Stigmata is the price of choosing your own nutrition. This is the story of her life and the reason she finally refuses to compete on their turf--but remains home-centered where her reality is in control.

AVERSION TO LUST AND AGGRESSION

Does the anorexic feel superior? Well maybe just more refined. Being thin she prefers privacy, and lust and aggression are terrible vulgar invasions of the fine. Her motto is "stay fine...stay free." In her primitive state she sought love to deal with family rejection, but when mature sees how it then turns destructive and controlling. As she becomes a lady with high boundaries it's "hands off". This defines the new Queen whose boundaries are very hard won. Overcoming sick relationships-used-as-emotional escapes while gaining strength and recovery through God is the precedent of success. The war-torn battleship often ends in celibacy which is marriage to the highest with no mortal infringement. Sex means officious invasion and distraction from the goal--her highest calling. As a priest once said, "celibacy is like a garden which after watering becomes more beautiful each day." She just wants to sleep (in readiness for the next day's hyper-creativity) when she hits the hay.

SEPARATION FROM FEMALE CULTURE

There's a herd (cultural conformity), then two sub-herds (male and female). There is far more allowance for uniqueness in the male herd while female culture is a massive impediment to genius. Feminists may say "women should get up, become, succeed". But once one does the hens begin to peck and peck to death. This dates back to paleo times as all through the centuries females compete for males—to be part of the "superior class". Female competition is a real and cruel thing and often the worst sexists are so-called "feminists." Am I being cruel here? Well like the notion of cruelty itself this is a veiled fact which may take a recovered anorexic to see. Suffice it to say that many ambitious women end up trusting only men as friends and their sisters the least of all.

PERCEPTIONS OF FROGS, PIGS OR HIPPOS

Loving God or a Gentleman and Nothing Less

To the stringently orderly anorexic encased in cerebrotonic peace and rigid diet restrictions the world seems a mess, a monotonous mistake, a monster. The frog symbolizes the "bed-hopper"--how easily they chum-up together! Social hall religion she will never understand: the world of banal, bothersome, busybodies seems out-of-touch with their own bodies and bloodstream.   They meet, they eat, they cheat, and while the body loses logic it becomes "loose": a lush, a leech, a lecherous lazy louse. Is she leery? Yes, so she makes lists and learns to love herself and the most refined, which is God or a Gentleman.

The pig is the epitome of swine consciousness, the opposite to self-restraint, let alone fasting. The hippo symbolizes the agitator who cannot leave well-enough alone. He gets a little restless and must hit, hate, harass and huff to make his presence felt. The hippo hates her hard-won and hallowed humming-along in her own stream. Does she hate people? No, she's only a realist who can only take the throne after forgiving it all.

The Dark Night of the Soul was felt by all Saints in history, just like Job. When in darkness never light your own fire through people, habit or food but just stop work, fast and wait on the Lord.

8

"NO!" and Turn

From Insanity, Insults and Intruders

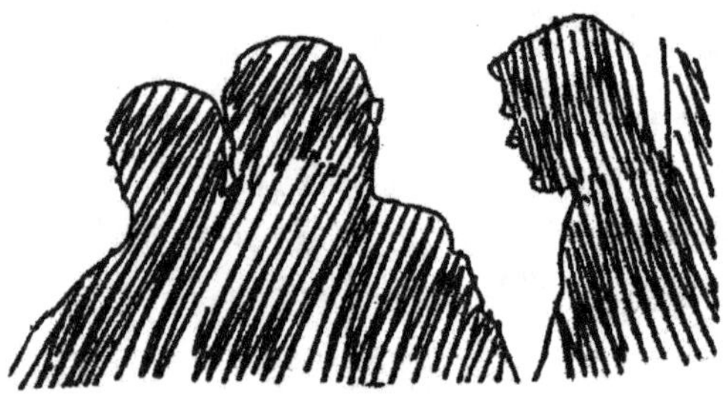

Look at those around you. These are the washed-out faces of "Yes-People". Howsoever God orders their steps they agree to their own demise by tolerating intrusion interrupting their plans. Having been taken away from the divine design they fall out of grace--the path of true success--and fail. But "NO" is like supplying electricity to a radio—a whole new world opens up as God fills your cup.

It's your life--adapt to none. Say "NO", turn from and repent. You must say no and then turn from distractions blocking success: people or habits. Everyone has a divine gift expressing God but few realize it--why? Because they are taken off their course by people and habits. The result: most never realize their goals as they tolerate tangents breaking their path. In this chapter you'll see what to eliminate to bring out your genius and the reward for what you love to do. Join the good life: with focused one-pointedness of mind your work gains glory in a life of abundance.

You've got gifts and talents from God and should only be pursuing those. Total commitment is needed to fulfill this call of God on your life. As you focus on this one thing it will be more anointed with God's power. But the world doesn't want that--it wants you to do its thing. The only way to fight the resistance is to stay centered until success.   Never let them steal your day so all your ways can be ordered rightly. You stay centered by learning to say "no", thus narrowing your focus and ordering your life instead of letting circumstances order you. The champions are single-minded and in control.

MESSERS

CHAMPION GUIDES

To mess means to make dirty and untidy, disarrange, bungle, interfere with, rough-up, meddle, manhandle, trifle. This is what happens with the interference of other people which can destroy your life and destiny, rob you of energy and take you out of grace. I'm talking to the would-be champions--your success is a delicate matter which must be handled like a crate of eggs--you must learn to say NO to hit the bull's eye. Stamp out distractions, for with all the competition out there, a near-hit is a huge miss. Find out what you do best and then just do that.

A good messenger is one who reliably bears a message or runs an errand. He brings good information upon which you may depend. A bad messenger is a bearer of evil tidings--he brings gossip against you, interferes with and tells you how to run your life. He encourages your confidences then leaks them out on the street. As you happily play a game alone, he arrives and changes it to suit him. He's a "messer" in confusion: you achieve structure and he takes you out of it. At this point you have a choice: stand up and be strong (say NO and do your work) or lay down and be weak (say YES and forget your goals).

YES PEOPLE

Millions suffer because they can't say NO. Just the word "NO" makes you King and Queen of your own domain. NO is the greatest power in the universe because it keeps you on course with God's power backing you up. NO keeps you on track, on top. Just think how many times your weak "Yes" lured you into trouble but NO--the sign of mature genius--always kept you safe. Image yourself saying NO to various requests--do it now: say "NO" twenty times. When "NO-ing" real situations the initial guilt will ease and as practice makes perfect it'll become fun as the release is felt each time. Simultaneously history will be seen with new eyes and you'll be aghast at your milquetoast personality of the past. The world is filled with crafty opposition to anything good like your Godly talents. The world wants your YES for their own gain, resulting in your loss. They want what is yours to be theirs. The weak end up giving it to them while the strong ignore them without a thought. The power of NO frees you from bother and intimidation wherever you go.

People use tricks to get your YES and prevent your NO. They make you feel guilty, disloyal, in danger. They promise, pretend, plead, persist, they shout and shock, they threaten, demand, rage, accuse, whine or weep. "NO" stops the tricks. NO is the highest form of intelligence backed up by God and the divine flow trying to come into your life. Users/ demanders want you to be theirs while God wants you to be free--to have all that is planned for you. Achieving this blueprint far exceeds anything you could ever plan for yourself.

NO leads you to an exciting new journey, to a happy land backed by the power to charge you up every single day. Think of why you say YES when you should be saying NO: fearing domination, relieving indecision, appearing friendly, because its easier than explaining, you've always said YES or they've promised rewards; because you want acceptance (more than your own life), everyone says yes or you fear angry reactions. Realize that it was just these timid tendencies that brought failure in your life.

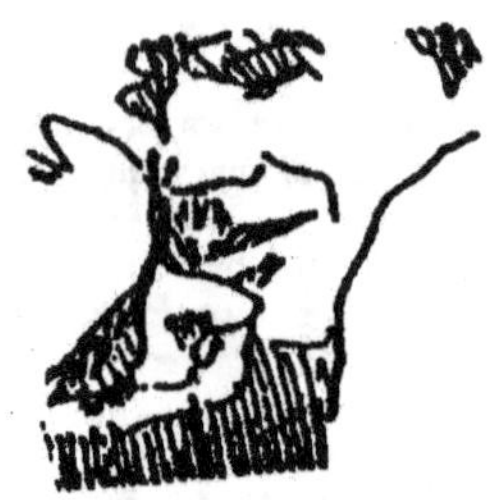

Looking back, YES created problems a NO could have avoided. Well now just say NO to the painful memories and learn your lesson. Like the world, painful memories try to drag you back into them--saying NO allows you to live in the total freedom of the present moment. The benefits are so great as NO becomes easier, that the guilt rising up soon disappears as you get your life back. Guilt from the world and the past is a trick of the lower self to keep you down. But you must never feel guilty about leaving a sleazy shack for a protected castle. Achieving your own fortified center in your home domain is like going from rags to riches.

LEARN TO ESCAPE

Learn to escape from your own self-defeat. Think of all the present situations where YES has to stop: Have you agreed to a monthly commitment that is really a burden? First realize the obstruction then just say NO--make the pertinent contact and resign, just like that. Forget all about your nervous timidity--do what is right to get your life back. Yes--your very life is the high calling of God, so the gold ring is at stake. Now that you have the information you must get the spiritual strength to apply it--yielding to God means NO, not YES! YES makes a mess and it always make you less. You are yielding to something higher than your own intellect through NO--permitting God and the spirit of truth to guide your life. This holy spirit gives total power to your NO just as electricity gives life to a radio. Its really the higher force that wants NO to reign, for it sees what is right in every circumstance then insulates—shuts things out--for your protection.

INVISIBLE SIGNALS

Everyone sends signals telling everything about them. Declaring strength through "no" keeps users away, for weakness (despondency, desperation) attracts them like flies. Only your signal of strength and command keeps plunderers at bay. These deceivers study you very carefully: While appearing casual they eye your every move, picking up cues from your dress, gestures, expressions. These are signals gauging their chances to score at your expense. Hoping for YES they poke and pry to test response, going as far as your weakness permits. Since every time the weak submits to the strong the formers "symptoms" come back, it is crucial to ask: is his business more important than mine, as his errands fall on me? From now on I will do what I want and feel peace!

9

GOD THE AVENGER

Repent Release and No Relapse—
and Revenge Comes Naturally

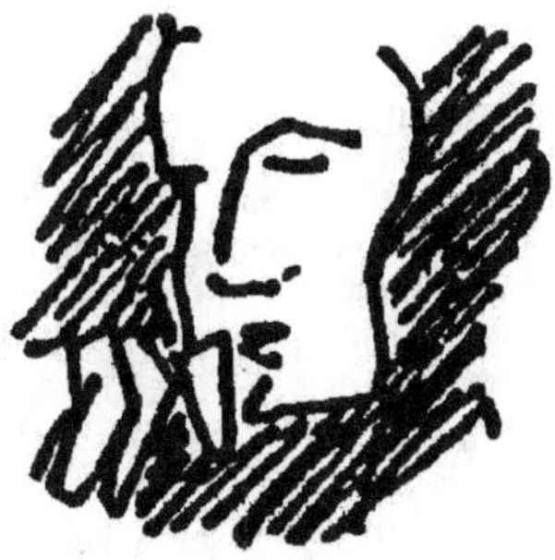

Everyone knows about terrible wars between countries--but there are also wars between siblings and silent ones between friends. We must win these wars and with God we can. He always avenges those who love Him, here on earth.

From the beginning of time it's always the same story: the herd sides against the Great. The champions, those with greatest potential, the ones God separates unto himself, those with the highest calling all are victims of the worst persecution. It's a mark of the Great! Once you understand this you'll take this tendency of human group nature as a compliment, as it indicates who you are. Let me ask you this: have you always felt you had something extraordinary in you, something that would later blossom to world success? Have you always felt you were meant to make an amazing new dent in this world? When you think of this vision does it always give you "high" hope? Then it is meant to be, for this is the mind of God in you.

Now let me ask you the second question--have people always sided against you as far back as you can remember? The answer is probably yes for they do indeed go together. It's just like the Biblical story of Joseph and his brothers. He had a vision of future greatness--which he dared to tell them in childhood-- and in return they jealously tried to kill him and sold him as slave. In fact, the life coming up to world success--the preparatory stage--is a major tough boot camp both because one is perfecting skills, character and walk with God but mostly because of the tremendous obstacles put there by jealous people.

HUMAN JEALOUSY
The Most Common Human Emotion

Your greatness excites tremendous envy and jealousy in people, and always has. This explains most all of your people problems. Especially if you be female, you likely felt jealousy coming from both sexes: women wanting to tear you down to be equal to them, and men wanting to use and conquer you--then pull you down to be beneath them. Overcoming these obstacles makes you so tough that you finally get like warm steel in your dealings with people--and this marks your readiness to reign. You must overcome the obstacles to creativity in dense herds before you can take the throne to work on removing these obstacles for all.

People siding against the great--take it as fate. Expect and prepare for it so you won't be hurt when it occurs (it's getting too late. You must always exit when seen as third-rate). The conformists become so weak minded they must group against you--you're too strongly independent! But if you stay close to God--your vindicator--nothing they can do will hurt you: you'll be safe under His wings. And God will avenge his own (those who love Him) so you have nothing to worry about--but when it's happening it can sure strike fear.

SYSTEMS THEORY AND INVERSION

Dealing with this terrible fear as the gang-ups occur is the last obstacle before success.   As you can see from the chapter on Anorexic Systems, the system set-up depends on the weakness in the parts--the identified patient whose very one-down position in the family system allows the others to play morally superior. Every sick system from the beginning of time needs a scapegoat onto which tension, conflict and the unacknowledged shadow is projected. As the "patient" begins to rise up and attain success the others react with violence or at least severe put-downs to regain the status quo with them on top. Her possible rise evokes a severe identity struggle in the others who have a huge investment in her scapegoat status. As she rises up, they react with accusations of her "cruelty" or "abuse" of them, her "protectors." It was only with her imminent success that a woman received this letter from her cruel abusive sister:

I'm finding it impossible to be around you anymore. Your abuse is overwhelming and can't take it anymore. No one else treats me with such disdain and disrespect and I don't have to take it anymore. You must get over your delusion and fantasy that you are an "author" and that you are going to publish your book. You have been deluding yourself for all of your adult life always claiming that it would be published in the near future. Of course we don't believe it but the sad thing is that <u>you</u> believe it.

This hurt very much but fortunately she knew about systems theory and that this was entirely predictable. Most happily she was soon published and these statements were untrue. That's the wonderful thing about completion--the lifelong sting-shots are now of none effect.

BE READY FOR ANGRY LOWMINDS

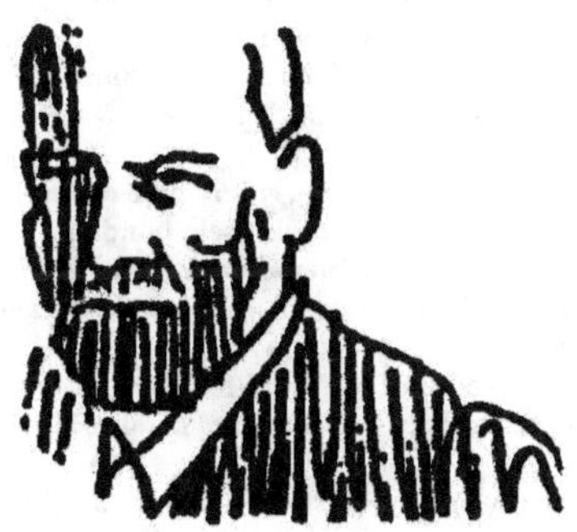

Having faith in the invisible even while thousands are against you will turn things around. It's just a test, so don't panic. God has to see the stuff you're made of before you can reign. Handling the inevitable persecutions coming from low-minds is part of this test. Enduring their gang-ups goes with the territory--it will always happen as the weak minds band together as one mind. Such is the contagion of madness, but one man can be a majority! You'll see--the fact that you're alone in this marks your superiority, and the fact that God has separated you unto Himself to do a job. Have faith in your solitariness and what it indicates--your getting stronger in these lessons.

Yes you must prepare for the mean actions of low-minds. This can make us angry as we are tested on forgiveness. Fighting back will only hurt you and increase their resistance. You must know God is the avenger and this fact should bring you great relief: If you avenge, God won't, but if you just stay sweet and wait, God will pour coals of fire on their head and reward you openly. They'll all know you're on top and will feel suddenly ashamed. I am dedicating this chapter to your great relief which is necessary for the saints. It's time you sensed the great justice of a God who protects his own, not in some "afterlife" but right now.

 Those who love God are protected by Him and He will surely go after the heathen tearing you (His beloved) down. I am now going to prove this to you by giving you a few Bible verses intended to trigger your aesthetic recognition of this occurrence throughout your life and the lives of others. They are so aptly and beautifully put you'll know it's God writing it and that He does what he says. As you look back over your life you will recall this happening just this way: You were in crisis as people bore false witness against you, and God took you through to Victory all hands down. Remembering these miracles will build great faith, the key to your continued success:

PSALMS ON GOD'S REVENGE

Blessed is the man who walks not in the counsel of the ungodly nor stands in the path of sinners nor sits in the seat of the scornful, but his delight is in the law of the Lord on which he meditates day and night...He shall be like a tree that brings forth its fruit in its season, whose leaf also shall not wither and whatever he does shall prosper...The ungodly are not so, but are like the chaff which the wind drives away...For the Lord knows the way of the righteous, but the way of the ungodly shall perish.

The Kings of the earth set themselves, and the rulers take counsel together, against the Lord and against his anointed saying "Let us break their bonds in pieces." He who sits in the heavens shall laugh--the Lord shall hold them in derision. Then he shall speak to them in His wrath, and distress them in His deep displeasure: "Yet I have set My King on My holy hill of Zion."   I will declare "You are my son-- today I have begotten you. Ask of me and I will give you the nations and the ends of the earth for your possession. You shall break them with a rod of iron, you shall dash them to pieces like a potter's vessel."

Lord, how they have increased who trouble me. Many are they who rise up against me...but I cried to the Lord and He heard me...I will not be afraid of ten thousands of people who have set themselves against me all around...Arise oh Lord, for you have struck all my enemies on the cheekbone: you have broken the teeth of the ungodly...for you alone Lord, make me dwell in safety...you shall destroy those who speak falsehood...the lord abhors the bloodthirsty and deceitful man....for there is no faithfulness in their mouth and their inward part is destruction...their throat is an open tomb...they flatter with their tongue...pronounce them guilty oh God. Let them fall by their own counsels.

But let all those rejoice who put their trust in you, because you defend them. For you O Lord will bless the righteous with favor. You will surround him as with a shield...my eye wastes away because of grief, it grows old because of all my enemies. Let all my enemies be ashamed and greatly troubled, let them turn back and be ashamed suddenly...Oh let the wickedness of the wicked come to an end, but establish the just--for the righteous God tests the hearts and minds. My defense is of God who saves the upright in heart. God is a just judge and God is angry with the wicked every day....He will sharpen his sword, he bends his bow and makes it ready. He also prepares for himself instruments of death--he makes his arrows into fiery shafts.

Behold, the wicked brings forth iniquity...he conceives trouble and brings forth falsehood. He made a pit and dug it out and has fallen into the ditch which he hath made. His trouble shall return upon his own head and his violent dealing shall come down on his own crown....out of the mouth of babes and nursing infants you have ordained strength because of your enemies, that you may silence the enemy and the avenger...when my enemies turn back they shall fall and perish at your presence. For you have maintained my right and my cause, you sat on the throne judging in righteousness. You have destroyed the wicked, you have blotted out their name forever and ever. O enemy, destructions are finished forever. And you have destroyed cities--even their memory has perished.

The Lord also will be a refuge for the oppressed, a refuge in times of trouble....when he avenges blood he remembers them...he does not forget the cry of the humble. Have mercy on me O Lord. Consider my trouble from those who hate me....Now the nations have sunk down in the pit which they made, in the net which they hid their own foot is caught...the Lord is known by the judgment he executes...the wicked is snared in the work of his own hands.

Suffice it to say the Psalms is all about overcoming persecutory enemies, and God saves His own. The mere fact that this dominates the most famous book in the Bible shows it's a pivotal part of the human condition and overcoming it a crucial part of coming into power--when we are given the nations to rule in our field. Your being alone makes them know you are great! Subconsciously we all know that to be set apart is sanctification. They may think "who do you think you are..." while they envy your independence and your high goals. Their hostility gets worse as they converse (with each other on the matter). You must be alone, for to be in their presence becomes a constant insult filled with sting-shots--that's how they command conformity: they want you on their turf so they can release conflicted energy at your expense.

RECAP

Just hold on, for your victory is soon and sure. You reach a point in completion where destiny takes over and even you can't stop your success. The foundation has been laid and now God takes over to complete His work through you. You've sown the seeds and now harvest time is here. Take your eyes off the past pain and persecutors--they can't hurt you now, but your fear they can will trip you up. Just remember regarding your war: it's God's battle so you won't even have to fight. If you have that faith, success is sure. Faith in God's vengeance is a must. When down in fear, read this section over and over again. You must believe in your victory, but first you must know there is a war. Then you will pray for victory so God can take you there. To return to the story of Joseph, once he became the King of Egypt his brothers feared his reprisal but Joseph acted like nothing happened and forgave them totally. Whether your weapon is writing, waiting on God or just working on Self the inversion of systems will occur now--enantiodromia will open up your whole new world with you on top for once.

10

PSYCHE OF SENSUALITY

Escape Sin and Systems and Joy's Made Full
—This is Sensual, the Only Bridge to Paradise

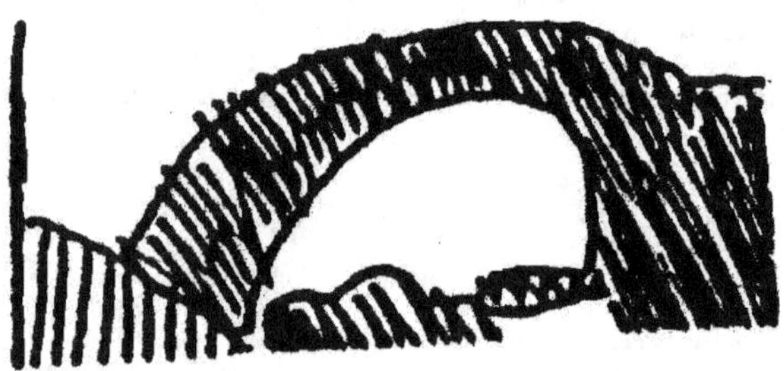

THE MEAN MOODS OF MAN

The mean moods of man--they all come from sin. The Bible says "Is there wrath amongst you? Then there is sin." If we can accept this fact right off the bat we'll have sidestepped much futile debate and get on with it--these mean moods are coming from sin which we should confront the mere appearance of. Once you've crossed that mental bridge, nip it in the bud! But usually words won't work--silent fasting is an automatic perfection so that enantiodromia (system inversion) can now occur. To put your life in perfect order never agree with evil by succumbing to the warped requests of humans (never degrade to adapt). Only upgrade others by becoming beautiful and never forcing the fit to them again. Just your new transformation will force them up instead.

There are two nervous systems, two sides to the brain. The two systems align with two perceptual styles: active (tunnel-vision) vs. receptive (wide-angled diffuse). The hot pursuit of pleasure (pleasure-seeking) is often a compulsive, active tunnel-vision which prevents true pleasure. This real joy only exists in the receptive mode which is non-compulsive, relaxed and diffuse. In contrast,   pleasure-seeking is only compulsive as it spills over to other people through persuasion and manipulation.

ACTIVE-RECEPTIVE MODES

I see a delicious difference between the active and receptive modes. After a long day of work (tunnel-vision) I seek the receptive--a direct switch in which everything like music is experienced differently and new thoughts rise up. My life has improved remarkably by knowing the difference and purposely switching between the two states of work vs. leisure. For a writer, leisure is the most important for compulsive, impatient action will always lose because true insights only arise in relaxation. The receptive mode is true sensuality, while the active mode becomes--or comes out of--a state of sin. Since this compulsivity is out of grace the results can be devastating while in the receptive mode they are joyous and productive.

SERPENT COILS TIGHTER: ENERGY MISAPPLIED

Every time we give into a pleasure-device to avoid anxiety the serpent winds tighter in a trap--the device becomes a vice of bondage. Sin is always repetition: energy recycled in outworn channels. As the years go by in this tunnel-vision which neurophysiologically cannot bring true pleasure, the sin becomes more entangling and more automatic until one is blind to its killing effects. The anxiety and bad memories it intends to hide are only more inflamed and distorted as addiction becomes a loss of reality.   An example is anorexic-bulimia which has little to do with food but rather the repression of feelings which are "stuffed down." Eating does that so well it becomes a huge trap which gains a life of its own: a solid blind addiction.

The more energy one has at birth the more energy is channeled to addiction—misapplied energy—and the more tremendous the release with repentance. Repent to become a rare dynamo. Then you have mastered the one thing the "he-man" or social "she-woman" never could--the mastery of the instincts. The same applies to sex. How interesting that sex and food are the two instincts justified by the present culture: "do whatever you want--no rules or restrictions." Rebellious at authority, people hate all rules yet the champions know the rules apply for the highest reason--total victory in dense herds.

ESCAPE THE TRAP

The sinner needs the fix more but enjoy it less. The addict must have the fix, so morals degrade in the attempt to get more. Because it is used to avoid, life is unimaginable without it and as one is weakened by this loss of reality the ego must compensate for the loss and selfishness sets in—the addict becomes untrustworthy. Now we see how ridiculous it is to read psychology books or see therapists while not repenting of sin. William James in varieties of religious experience remarked how the "symptoms" leave with repentance. Releasing the addiction brings an explosive transformation as the serpent, made stronger each time one gave in, unwinds and shoots up the spine in a spiraling release of energy. This release brings tremendous creativity as the obstructive ego is dissolved. Giving up addiction brings a pink cloud and beautiful vista: extreme joy unimaginable when in the addicted state needing a fix. Only the strong can enjoy true pleasure of the senses and only the weak get hooked in order to avoid. This is the sequence in the lives of humans from the beginning of time: give up sin, and the symptoms leave!

TRUE VS. FALSE PLEASURE

True pleasure is omnipresent, since it's enjoyment exists in the experiencer himself. In the relaxed, leisurely receptive mode it's all pleasurable and no one thing takes dominance. In contrast to the active pursuit of pleasure, no one thing binds the personality into perversion which is the opposite to just feeling the pleasure every moment--of being alive and enjoying the elements of sun, moon, stars, angels, times of day, seasons, tastes, sounds, aromas, prayer and pleasant company. Moreover, the pleasure of interacting is different from the addictive social-climbing and socializing to be "seen." Most of all pleasure-seeking in this culture is active, which is why obesity is the leading disease--it is active eating to avoid which holds the person bound.

Many divorced women stick their head into a refrigerator, balloon-up and never come out. Once eating is associated with soothed emotions it becomes an insuperable stronghold in the personality. When the same old hurts rear up the food-force is far greater than the person herself. Bad character develops when in the grips of the emotion-eating demon for one does anything and neglects everything to serve it. The addictive loss of reality which is tunnel-vision serves only the bruised ego. This results in the jungle mentality of shooting and shadows and always looking for ways to maintain the addiction through deceit and covering one's tracks.

ONLY RECEPTIVITY IS PLEASURE

The receptive mode is ecstatic continuous pleasure. But it cannot be maintained if there is contradiction and duplicity in the personality--for these alert the system for emergency, automatically throwing it into tunnel-vision. The weak addict is "busted, disgusted and cannot be trusted." His grasping nature becomes as intense as his desire to escape the pain of inevitable rejection and persecution, and his fear of losing the fix means other people are again used and abused. The more weak, the more grasping. The more warped, the more tragic his mistakes. Here a stronghold has developed--an area out of the will of God, dictated only by damaged ego. It is blocked energy in the thought-life and this means lost success and ruin.

What a relief—one has made gold by going through the fire, the addiction is gone and he enters the receptive mode: like a huge jigsaw puzzle beautiful pieces of life now come together miraculously. This synchronicity is an intense enjoyment of each piece, not holding on to any one part but going from one pleasure to another: the pleasure of the morning, the pleasure of finishing chores, the pleasure of a drive, the pleasure of working in the garden or chatting with the neighbors. We enjoy one pool of activity at a time. Moderation is the key--the "high" in all good things.

RECEPTIVE MODE AND INNER JOURNEY

So many good things--why over-spend time with any one of them? Enjoy each pool, then go on to another. This gives fascination, variety and energy to life. The key is high energy (from non-addiction) which brings jubilance and constant surprises: welcome to the life of phased highs--in which we are intensely in the moment, not nervously trying to avoid the past or future with the fix. The psychology of sensuality refers to two things: (1) the right-brain relaxed normal love of pleasure which becomes a continuous appreciation of life itself, and the (2) grasping, addictive, left-brained tunnel-visioned pursuit of pleasure to avoid pain or anxiety which becomes a trap as the pain gets worse resulting in a distortion of reality and perversely bad character.

One can be addicted to anything and there is nothing that cannot be addicting. People are the worst addiction, the most all-consuming--yet the Bible says "trust no man." Good relationships are established through time and testing. Be patient and cease chumming up casually, for great caution is the order of the day--exclusivity. Avoid the opposite (the people fix) for inclusion is incaution--though politically correct inclusion will bring your ruin!

SELFISHNESS

All addicts are selfish--they're so self-consumed they literally can't think of anyone else. Being insensitive they say indiscrete things: these are autonomisms which are part of addiction and beyond control. Are they intentionally cruel, dense and grossly negligent or just addicts? It's the biological instincts (food and sex) that become compulsive traps of lower desire--quick-to-shoot carnal temptations. They bring pleasure (temporary relief) but each time one "gives in" the serpent wraps tighter and the bad memories become more warped. At this point development into maturity is arrested for we don't grow if cemented into addictive tunnel-vision. Whether high-class doctor, wealthy female CEO or president of the United States one remains a baby. We can't be ladies and gentlemen just by wanting to--we are what we are. The tiger doesn't change its spots--only inner work brings transformation of the person. It is beautifully summed up by this pastoral letter to a wife regarding her unfaithful husband:

Dear Hillary:

What you're going through is so common. Things broke down in the sixties and now we see the despicable culmination. Men are so influenced by prevalent pornography and perversion. I was shocked by his shameless talk of sex. A Godly man has class--refinement and respect. It's the difference between the dignified old movies and the sick sex-filled and slovenly new ones. The world is now filled with dirty old men and loose women. I pray he'll achieve the refinement of a man his age. And what of your daughter: children develop such high tolerance for these sick situations they lose discernment and marry the same type under the same denial. It's the "polygamous spirit" which hits middle-aged men--these aging baby boomers can be arrogant, greedily thinking they deserve two or more women to abuse. If women adapt rather than confront bad character the abuse worsens as man's self-hate projects back onto them. For the sake of your family keeping a moral household is crucial.

For don't think your girl doesn't sense something's wrong--though not putting her finger on it evil has a psychic stench which is always followed by depression...

THE END TIMES: MEN ARE

The superior man is in conflict with the petty negative forces trying to pull him down to something they can understand. His job is to develop the moral strength to overcome these resistances to creativity and rise up to make an amazing new dent in the world. To do this he must repent of sin for without this he can't have the necessary boldness and confidence to make a dent. The Bible says in the end times men are self-loving, money-loving, arrogant, profane, malicious gossipers, unrestrained, brutal and vicious haters of good, treacherous, conceited, religious in form but really unholy, captivating of weak women and always learning but never coming to the truth.

It is very difficult to live in this generation. Hi-tech progress camouflages the severe degeneration in other areas: mind, spirit, body, family and knit of society. As society degrades so too the individual as the herd maintains its feeble cohesion through strict conformity ("politically correct thinking") which is a mass resistance to true genius. As people degenerate together they become "dull normal."

A CHAMP AMONGST SHARKS

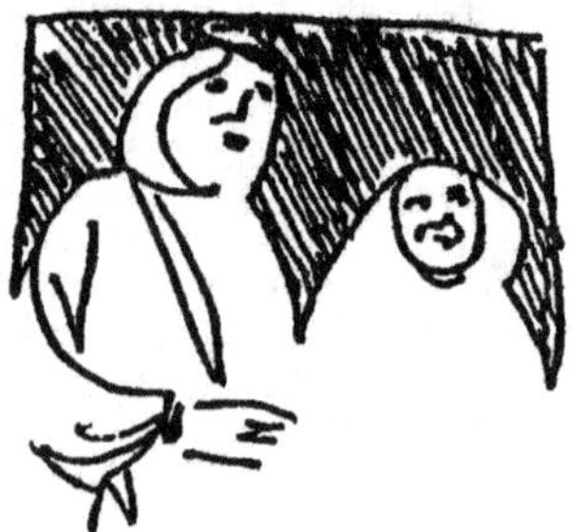

The superior man is a champion standing out as a shining angel in a sea of sharks. He must show a brilliant radiant life reflecting God--making spirit-based decisions not on what the majority thinks, logic, uncalled-for advice of neighbors or "common sense." He is not led by puny, finite, darkened minds of men but inspired by the infallible inerrant laws of God--the ones that Jesus knew and Einstein proved. Deal with these times by becoming sensitive to nature, love, beauty and genius. Note the futile lives of the ungodly—vanity, carnality, misery. While keeping your own calm, poise and righteousness it helps to realize (but not relapse because of) the mean moods of men and women who are still stuck.

THE PSYCHE OF SENSUALITY

CHAMPION GUIDES

People clamor for the psyche of sensuality thinking it's about sex rather than the consequences of sin which are real. Since the punishments are inherent in the sin itself, repentance will bring a metamorphosis beyond belief! The Bible says to the champions: "go out and take the land." But to do this we must be bold and courageous as we tell the simple truth. One can never have this courage while in sin which brings discouragement. If in sin we lose that power, in a spirit of fear veiled by compensations like hype and spin. To be bold, we must have the self-love coming from purity. Sin makes us weak, creating more cravings for sin to "fix things."

AVOID THEIR FACES

Most people refuse to act before they "look at their faces" to discern approval and disapproval. They value "their" response to determine worth and value, as if the herd is any barometer! Grow up--you'll be OK if you don't look at their faces. You must now preach and teach with a bag over your head--never be dismayed at the fear of man lest God let you be overcome. If God says you can succeed, you can! One's only problem is the fear of people for when fear is chosen over boldness, lost faith fails to fit the fame and fortune God has planned for your future.

Be Bold. Be plain with the truth. Save the weak elements oppressed by the powerful—that is, the dominant view. Living in the past or fearing mass rejection puts us ever-under pressure. This pressure comes from sin, for weakness teams with the majority who is out-of-grace. The pressure from sin is endless, so baby-boomers should wake-up and tell the truth. Don't let evil stand, pray for divine vindication and know your foes! Perhaps you should recognize who they are first--for degradation, gossip or treachery is no sign of friendship.

SIN IS AMNESIA, PURITY IS TOTAL RECALL

Everything we experience is stored in the five senses. Nothing is "forgotten"--it's all there but inaccessible until we're clear. A witness of an accident can't recall the license number of the culprit until hypnosis brings it all up--even though he can't remember seeing it in the first place. When in sin we're blinded to even the obvious--this is denial. Repentance allows experience to double, triple, increase by tenfold, one hundred-fold: all blinders are dropped and the floodgates are laid bare! And thus the fast is a vision quest as all information—past, present and future--is recalled to mind. A cleansed bloodstream or sudden freedom from oppression (from mind or man) brings it all out. Repenting of so-called "pleasures" opens us to more pleasure, a veritable phantasmagoria never experienced before. The promise is: once clean you'll wonder why you waited so long as you float blissfully in the arms of God. Welcome to true experience and real energy!

Let us pause in life's pleasures and count their many tears. Hard times, hard times—come again no more. Willie Nelson

11

AGELESS CORNUCOPIA

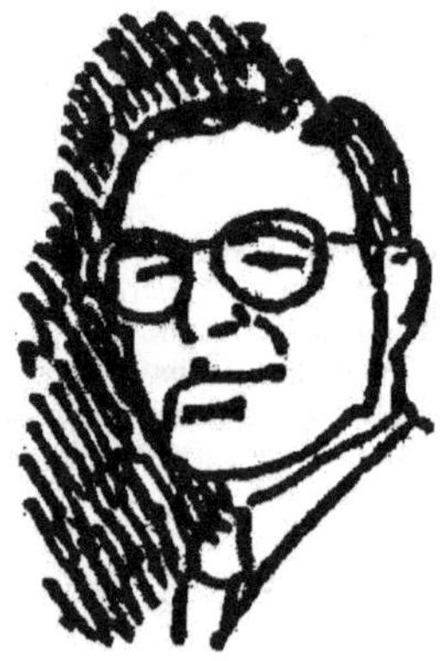

This chapter is for the elders and all the young people who fear aging. Take joy--there is nothing to fear, only much to look forward to. As the brain expands in old age the temporal lobe opens up to eternity and ecstatic witness. End all fears--the future is only fullness with our culminating perfection at life's end (our highest blend).

It's a sick culture that puts down the older generation through the glorification of youth. It's not only unfair, it is false because old age is the culmination of life, a crown of glory and a time of heightened mental development. The temporal lobes burst open to reveal eternity, and thus eternal wisdom can only be gained from the mentorship of the elder. We should look forward with glee due to the facts you are about to see. Everything you have been told--every fear-laden myth you have swallowed whole--is false, for the elder is mentally superior in the sagacious jubilee. The time of life when physical powers wane mark the beginning of the magnification of mental powers. It is the fact that we don't know this while simultaneously allowing a sick culture to tell us the opposite which creates the degeneration we see all around. An ageist culture is a sick culture.

VISION QUEST INTO ELDERHOOD

The Vision Quest is an ancient Shamanic rite of passage in which the seeker retreats from civilization, goes to a sacred place in nature and cries for a life vision of purpose. I took this Vision Quest twenty years ago by leaving society to live in a small desert cabin on 230 acres of wilderness. This was the happiest time of my life, in total solitude and natural beauty. I loved the seasons, the times of day and sharing this beauty with five dogs and a cat. I spent these years in solitude, fasting, prayer, meditation, writing, studying, biking, working in the yard and taking long walks. I entered an entirely new reality.

It was a transition from the old to the new life--an initiation into elderhood, or becoming a sage. By individuating into completion I was preparing early for elderhood but by previously clinging to youthful things I was avoiding completion, the thing I wanted most. It wasn't until I saw elder mysticism—"eldering"--as an inner journey that I understood human aging as a wonderful culmination which should naturally get better until the very end.

SICK CULTURES HATE "OLD"

This culture shows a deep-seated fear and loathing of old age, which should be the greatest time of life. Due to the baby boom the elders are the fastest-growing segment of America with 76 million. The age wave is a tidal wave, yet it comes at a time when ageism is most intense. To offset ageism the boomers had better understand that aging is harvest time, the culmination of a lifetime of lessons and the true party. They should see aging as the badge of success it is, a time of unparalleled inner growth--for only at harvest time do we gain the panoramic vision essential to lead the tribe. Thus the elder is invaluable to the race, not a liability to it.

People enter old age with fear and trembling. Feeling betrayed by their bodies and defeated by life they expect to suffer from reduced enjoyment, vigor and usefulness. Their plight is made far worse by the trivialization and minimization by society and family—the signs are all around that they are obsolete, of no value. How sad and how false. The elders are wisdom-keepers for society's well-being by opening up magnified intelligence transmitted as legacy. This joy crowns an elder's life with worth and nobility. Have you ever noticed their uncanny psychic powers? They see through walls, they're our wake-up calls! The notion of sage or elder should replace all negative images while giving us all something to look forward to. "Eldering" will release tremendous vitality and vigor into the peak of our life. It will be for me, as I see a life of work coming to its culmination and reward. For the mature, old age is the opposite to bored—for all through history it was the last phase when the saint's spirit soared.

Aging is not the problem. The problem is the cultural images which tragically guide our lives into fear and panic. If we have models which are positive, healthy and active we can dramatically expand into a mysterious adventure as we go forward. Only this time of pure inner richness grows sages healers and prophets—it's the most important time of life!

LESS MATTER, MORE SPIRIT

It is physical decline which awakens this elder consciousness of expanded powers. It is precisely the loss of one which elicits the other. Let's explore this further, for consciously embracing aging early triggers the process of individuation and completion (eldering) while avoiding the pitfalls of later becoming "elderly." The breakdown of the youthful body leads to the breakthrough of the elder's higher consciousness. And so elderhood arises in the context of decline: When the psyche issues a call to engage in life completion, matter lessens to maximize energy and spirit. Less matter, more spirit! It's the icing on the cake, the celebration, the party after a life of labor, pain and utterly being controlled by other people. Why? Because less is more!

In old age we heal relationships and our pasts, enjoy our achievements and leave a legacy. The elder can bless all the triumphs and tragedies he came through and re-frame the dreams, disappointments and betrayals into wisdom. The meaning of the play will now become clear in elderhood, the crowning achievement.

NO ROLE MODELS

The culture provides no models for aging, so we're all uncomfortable with it. In contrast, "elder sagacity" or mysticism—eldering--rediscovers old age as an achievement to savor and enjoy. Postmenopausal women who feel invisible in a youthist culture will suddenly become radiant as they release deep-seated tensions. Rather than remorse over the past, the elder recontextualizes his past through panoramic vision, reframing past mistakes to "mine" them for wisdom.   The result is a peace, and this is power! If we avoid distracting (and comparatively boring) worldly amusements and just contemplate we gain a peaceful goldmine of invention and wit as ageist stereotypes are replaced by a deja-vu of coming attractions.

We're all so starved for models that even knowing an expanding elder infects us with enthusiasm. It's like entering the senior year in excited anticipation of attaining the high values we all crave. Having grown beyond the drive for personal power, a deeper humanity emerges as harvesting and deep reflection gives us our place in the cosmos.

CLING TO YOUTH OR SELF-COMPLETION?

Having no models we either fall into depression and decline or strive to compete with youth. But if we view age as the gold summit, we feel something very special growing inside and nourish it to harvest the gold. We can't stay hooked to rushing around and conquering. Women must drop youthful seduction to attain higher standards: the dignity of elder beauty—thus reclaiming the right to age without stigma!

CHAMPION GUIDES

When elders identify with early works or looks they end in conflict. The deep psyche urges us to harvest our lives, not obsess with the outer world. Staying stuck makes us prey to sadness, bitterness and defeat. Instead just enjoy this sacred stage: relax, listen to the inner voice, take naps! All our lives we conformed and catered to the convenience of other people, not the promptings of the inner life. Society completely ignores our bio-relationship to nature so grow up--go within. Living to the ebb and flow of this strong force is like ocean going through the veins--this is your own inner nature, so take the reins! First contemplate, then decide your new agenda for the last and greatest season of life—for the fine finale may even be flamboyant fame and fortune.

ACHIEVEMENT OK, ENJOYING NO-WAY

Our culture schools us on achieving, but not enjoying the fruits of our labor. We were never taught that enjoyment was enough. Instead it's always more--more pleasure, travel, possessions or relationships. We need the help of mysticism to cultivate calmness and contentment, for this breaks attachments to the social persona in order to reclaim the True Self we abandoned to socially adapt. Aging is really a natural monastery stripping away these phony roles, attachments and pleasures and what emerges is a miraculous sense of discovery and new energy transcending "doing" in favor of "being." These are the gifts of contemplative old age and I for one aim to enjoy this phase way before it hits. Fearing it is the pits for on this hard-won pinnacle wisdom sits.

YOUTH: NO TIME TO CONTEMPLATE

When young one is just too busy to cultivate this quiet inwardness spawning mystical experience. To please society youth must put the inner journey on hold, shirking contact with the sacred to master skills instead. Elderhood reconnects to the sacred and takes the universe back in. Rid of demanding and restrictive roles its like loosening a tight-fitting costume and slipping into cozy pajamas. I now see naps as the most productive thing I could do, for the higher brain is recharging. Having finally become individualized we are entitled to do our own thing without adapting to anyone else's standards. What a wonderful period of life--only the rich can afford this life of leisure when young!

ELDERS MUST SPEAK OUT

Once whole the elder's duty is to infuse the public with higher values, like telling the powers-that-be they should be ashamed behaving like children playing games of dominance. As world-mother you'll see extraordinary things as people bow down showering you with gifts. That's how starved they are for role models. As you transcend silly fears you'll grow to full stature and speak out with greater authority. At your age you're sure of your highest identity and beliefs--so speak publicly. Just hold your head up high and tell the simple truth, for to cower before youth is simply uncouth. Become a sage—they'll line up to your booth.

As elders speak from the authority of the God-made True Self, something wonderful occurs. Listeners re-discover inner knowing--that heart knowledge that links them to nature and the world. As elders speak, armor drops and thus they maintain the consciousness of the whole tribe. When youth turns to the elder they are yearning for something more--that vast unexplored territory residing in a sage who is only now peaking in old age. When old we can create a destiny from choice, not expectations.

ELDERING IS TRUE SUCCESS

Elderhood is a great success. The sage is charged with the evolutionary task of guiding society--what a joy, we deserve it! You must inspire society to replace it's shortsighted bottom-line mentality with the natural: spirit, nature and God. As sage-ing takes root in your heart you'll see a glorious future awaiting you, no matter what your age. It's when the physical fades that the fire alights from within until in our eighties we become most passionate, intense, flaming with a wild life beyond expression--a swelling clarity that expands into lives with passion and mystery. Our spirits will be questing, not resting. Our consciousness will grow, not slow. Elderhood is a quantum leap into the second life of spiritual realization.

LIFE STARTS AT SIXTY

Sixty plus is God's gift to humanity. No need to compete and be "liked." Un-caged energy releases into pure capacities restrained in youth. No time for trivia--we begin to create. Sages balance the inward ascetic with the outward human by expressing the True Spirit in the mundane world whose only hope is growing beyond the materialism which is only misery.

We are the culmination of a huge life process. If we unfold we open to incredibly higher being: the secret, mysterious, unique greatness of the True Self seeking expression. If in a nurturing environment with just God or other expanders we will experience a brain spurt linked to spirit. This happens in adolescence but emerging sexuality smothers it--then such a spurt into higher evolution is mistaken for libido and the spiritual is misplaced into sexual/social channels. The spiritual quest goes underground until now in elderhood.

MIND SHARPENS AS BODY DECLINES

Old age is a fascinating and exciting time of exploration, mysterious adventure and spiritual discovery. As the body gets tired the mind gets sharper. The challenge is to risk all frames of reference and outer props opening the mind to higher realms. Lifelong learning is the purpose of our species and when we stop we defeat the plan. Learning may peak in our late eighties when we contact a "giant spring" of skill, giving spectacular demonstrations, and the new habit of unlimited potential evokes new skills. With limitless possibilities we are open to constant surprise and anticipation--because of our age.

OTHER-DIRECTED LIFE WAS STRIFE

As you look back were you not lived by family, friends and fickle society? Were you not kept by jail-guards watching your every move? Did you not curtail your every natural expression, just to adapt? Did you not truncate parts of self just to fit in? What misery—I remember it well. Now we are self-directed flowering spirits in an inner search for God. By our detachment we promote a direct inner experience of Him and the divine. Conventional religion fills the need for social belonging but not necessarily contemplation and harvesting which reduces the ego as it opens the spirit. How different from the safe and secure social-religious identity--without access to the real depths people cling to religious brand-names, past fames and mind-games.

CELLS   REJUVENATE

Through the inner journey cells are rejuvenated and aging is retarded. If operating as usual--in superficial, social and secular thinking--we speed up the aging of cells. But as we move to the silent transcendent, mental activity stops and cells revive. I can sure feel this change when relaxing after a stressful work or social situation. Solitude in silence brings this instant shift to the revelatory rewards of the right-brain. From too much "left" the elder must refrain, or become insane.

Those dismissed as "old" are actually agents of human evolution, for throughout history the elder symbolizes the unique flowering of humanity: a rare once-in-a-time event. In India the sage functions as father confessor and spiritual guide. These flowering sages have revelations and peak experiences we can all have when older: mystical perception, creative inspiration, scientific discovery, invention and extrasensory perception.   Intuition is nonlinear, bringing together simultaneous fields in knowledge and perception—leaping way ahead of slow-moving logic by showing the "big picture" instead.   This instantaneous knowing brings the contagion of joy, whereas everyday logic deadens like lead.   Everyday man is concerned with what someone "said" while the psychic-intuitive sage gives them simple truth so they're truly fed.

GREAT ARTISTS DO BEST AT 90

History shows many elders producing great works of beauty and science in later years. Frank Lloyd Wright did his greatest work at seventy, Picasso at 90. Freer air blows in later years--what joy and vitality when free of society (no more tears). The stakes are less, intimidating jailers are gone and there are new reserves in courage, wisdom and open fields of experiment. The creative life is far more possible later as intuition connects us to the natural environment: a much higher life, free of strife--the power of God's wife. Yes God will support you with power and energy—if free of human society—for He knows you are physically weaker while having His work to do. More power is infused into a Majority of One because you're not with crew. How to get to God's power: become weak. Through you just let Him speak, for he always gives energy where needed (without leak).

ELDER   BRAIN   EXPANSION

The most primitive brain is the reptilian, dealing with basic survival--it is territorial and habit-driven. The next area is the limbic brain which relates us to the social world--it is rhythmic (hypnotic), ritualized activity hooking us to the herd. The third layer is the neocortex of intuition exploding suddenly into communion with God. It is the social world and habits (we use to distract us from aging) that prevents the opening of this marvelous goldmine.

The frontal lobes of the neocortex have highest intuition, creativity and a cornucopia of magnified perceptions awaiting the elder who opens to it. This interior universe is vast and infinite. Moreover, the temporal lobes of the neocortex are associated with paranormal and psychic experiences. But if you drag the past into the present you'll be impervious to the fulfillment, vitality and pure delight of your increasing unfoldment. No matter what age the expanding elder faces the future optimistically. But if at eighty his consciousness is stuck at 40 he'll stagnate and suffer a haunting despair. Be advised, for you see it all around—from their hearts and minds no sound, like their only hope is beneath the ground!   There is no wisdom here, only confound.   Their only thoughts are of the past, when big in town.

BOOMERS FIXATED BY YOUTH
That's So Uncouth

Although baby boomers have grown through meditation, when it comes to aging they're still fixated by youth culture. It's to these peers that I speak: It's so dangerous clinging to youthful things--it prevents the sagacity to lead the tribe and individuate, the whole meaning of eldering. Thanks to natural diet and exercise, boomers are the fastest-growing elder group in America and the over-sixties are growing twice as fast as the rest of the population. So become an enlightened sage when older, the esteemed member of your growing tribe! Talk to youth, but especially to peers—make them seers, banishing fears, drying their tears. Tell them: "Evolutionary aging balances physical decline with mental flowering and skills--as one recedes the other blossoms" and watch their reaction (awesome).

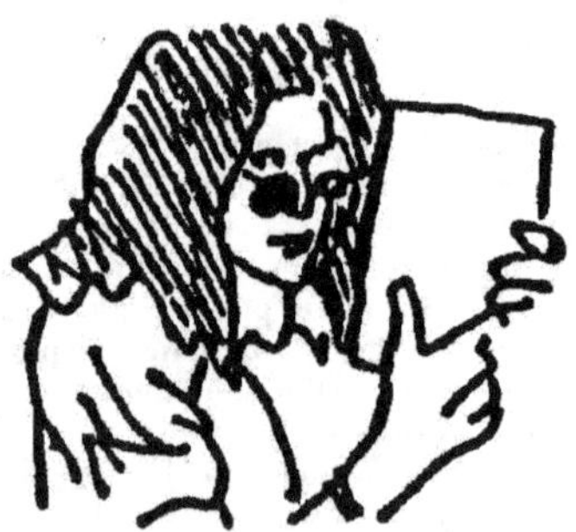

ELDERS ACROSS TIME AND SPACE

In America "old" is like being a leper. But in India "old" is an achievement of respect and recognition, as people cherish wrinkles and look forward to gray hair. Some exaggerate their age to gain greater respect, seeing old age as a time to detach from obligations and just ponder and enjoy. The Japanese see old age as a source of prestige with a national holiday called "honor the aged day." Native Americans see elders as wisdom-keepers safeguarding tribal survival.

The Bible is lavish in praise of elders as gray hair is a crown of glory and wrinkles a mark of distinction. "Thou shall rise up and honor the face of the old man." But the Greek world showed the gerontophobia (fear of age) from negative stereotypes that we see today. They valued youthful heroism, physical perfection and beauty--and aging was seen as a catastrophe and divine punishment. How myopic and tragic! Elder-status was raised in ancient Rome where their wise counsel carried great legal authority in the senate: "young men for action, old men for counsel." Cicero wrote "old age is respectable when it asserts itself and is not enslaved to any one. I admire a young man with an old man in him, and an old one with a young man in him--the man old in body but never in mind." To attain this state he must have "sound nutrition, exercise, sexual moderation and an active mental life of reflection." The bible-based Puritans saw old age as a sign of God's pleasure, divine election and a badge of supernatural sanctity. At New England town meetings it was not the rich but the elders who were given places of honor as repositories of knowledge and traditional values.

ELDERS ARE PATHFINDERS

Throughout history elders were the beloved pathfinders, luring us to old age in anticipation of powerful usefulness. Tribal elders made their imprint all through the Near East and Mediterranean cultures. To be called "old man" in ancient Israel was honored and wielded enormous religious and judicial power. To the ancients, old men were natural leaders using wisdom for problem-solving from the deep unconscious. The elders reveal our potentials— what can possibly be more important than that? With no models triggering these archetypal depths we are now lost in this world. Is it any wonder the degradation of morals, literacy and families—the utter hopelessness, drug addiction, divorces, fatherless homes? Society needs the elders to sustain it at its highest peak—the elders are the only check on certain degeneration.

TRADITIONAL AGING IS TRANSMITTING CULTURE

In primitive societies elders withdrew from everyday life to just think and transmit highest culture. But now, sadly, this social identity is stripped away and lost through "retirement". In literature we see the archetypal elder King Lear divested of power, living a wretched old age and descending into madness. Spiritual eldering provides the solution: an otherworldly celebrational spirituality, healing the split between spirit and matter and affirming sacred life—not the mundane, superficial, carnal materialism we see today. It's the difference between a boldly flamboyant array and the horror of old folk's homes (thinking that's "ok"). It's the difference between exciting life and optimistic anticipation of increasing unfoldment to the very end, and the terror of turning thirty—the current trend. Baby-boomers, unite! We are the majority so start the eldering revolution now—won't you, my friends?

TRADITIONAL CULTURES LOVE THE OLD

All the world's spiritual traditions have models of realized elders. The roshi in Zen, in Buddhism the lama, in Tibetan Buddhism the sheikh, in Islam the rebbe--all see aging as the phase of ultimate self-knowledge. For the Hindus, four ashramas map the changing spiritual needs of the human life cycle, culminating in the True Self and service to society. So the Indians think of life as a four-stage spiritual journey: Brahmacharya: gaining the intellectual and moral tools for adult life. Grihasta: marrying, having children, being social and working for wealth. Vanaprastha: detaching from family and social identity to pursue the spiritual. And in the final stage sannyasa one transcends all limited identification with family, religion, race and nation. As wondering single renunciates they become citizens of the world devoted to self-realization, spiritual teaching and selfless service to society. We can remain in family and community and still detach from social roles and deepen the contact with God. Do it and receive love from a nation famished for elder models!

THE INNER JOURNEY OF ELDERING

Today we see the ageism of ancient Greece, every bit as offensive and dangerous as racism and sexism. It discourages the elder influence, so like any downtrodden group they sequester into retirement communities to commiserate together and strengthen their shoddy identity. The movement called "successful aging" sees the solution in physical health but leaves out the spiritual altogether: In a one-sided drive to alter, reverse or control the aging process it just impoverishes it more by trying to "restore youth" rather than appreciating aging as a wonderfully superior stage of the human experience. The only solution is the inner journey! Go inside, ride the tide and become cosmic, bonafide.

IT SHOULD BE EASY
Not Make Us Queasy

Because we are not contemplative in our productive years, many face a painful abyss in unstructured retirement. Let's see retirement as the Indians do: a spiritual vocation while being on vacation--something prepared for in middle age by becoming contemplative, artistic, studious, sensitive and gentle. Seek this and you'll be supported from both our own depths and on high. As we detach from social and professional identities the whole universe rushes in to support our "No" answers while "Yes" brings relapse into old ruts. By doing inner work when young we won't disorient or panic when outer props go later, and   thank God they do! For we're brand new--past props can't enter the stew. This wonderful apex must remain true, fearlessly and powerfully with God through-and-through. Does this not thrill you too?

HARVESTING IS WONDERFUL

In traditional cultures harvesting a life in old age is easy, but in ours it is painfully difficult. Harvesting means: gathering the fruits of a life and enjoying them. It can be from within as quiet self-appreciation or without through honor, respect and recognition. But without eldering consciousness our own gerontophobia destroys the harvest. The cure-all is to exchange secular for sacred power—making us shamans, healers and priests. In the new context of aging, elders have a wild almost prankster-like quality which sees the humor in all situations. Like Buddha they laugh at everything they see or think! This new reality is like going from shabby cotton to mink, but only if elders are respected (not rejected) do they stay in the pink.

ELDERING IS COSMIC TRANSFORMATION

Carl Jung developed elder psychology in terms of individuation, the process of becoming the complete human being of our destiny. In the afternoon we can't live by morning's program but rather turn inward to reconnect with the self which was silenced by our social slots or slovenly sins. This revealed cosmic being is our personal center speaking through dreams, visions and images. A human being would not grow to 70 or eighty if longevity had no meaning for the species--later life has great significance of its own, not merely a pitiful appendage. Whoever carries youth into old age pays through soul-damage, for spirituality must take precedence when energy wanes and friends and family are lost. It's the spiritual outlook cure—so make the grandkids call you ma'm and sir! And never envy youth (the false lure) for despite the glorified image there is much trouble there (in this evil age it's often impure). You are much better off here, in the radiant cosmic elder tour.

LIFE IS EIGHT TURNING POINTS

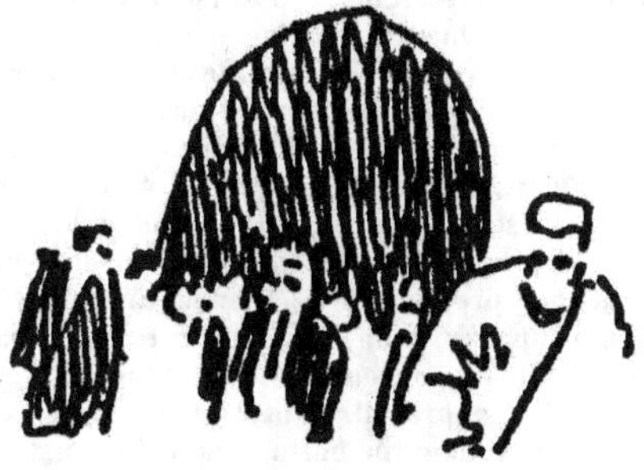

Erik Erikson saw life as a sequence of eight turning points which can turn to good or bad results. Resolving each step leads to new growth and maturity while failure at any point ends in neurosis and stunted growth at that level. In the final stage of ego integrity vs. despair, completion and self-acceptance is achieved—and it is this which offsets the physical decline. Wisdom is the acceptance of our one and only life as something which had to be by necessity and permitted no substitutions. And to think we spent our lives in shame and self-doubt for the very destiny that had to be! Acceptance without shame makes us handsome, ageless blueprints made by God, while shame and guilt makes us aging deformities—a clod.

FAIRY TALES AND ARCHETYPES

Fairy tales give insights into youth and elder psychology, reflecting the different concerns of the emerging growing personality: separating from parents, struggling for world placement, making commitments to spouse and career. The elder tales symbolize the tasks of the second half of life: not growing old but of growing through transcendence and knowledge of self and God. Elder tales begin with the old man in isolation and barrenness. Then by miracle he rediscovers the magic: by accepting his losses of family, friends, fickle society and it's "fun" he is transformed as he confronts issues repressed since youth--the dark unknown side called the shadow. As he breaks free of society and faces this shadow he gains "emancipated innocence." He comes together whole an ageless child--by having faced what he had always denied and by detaching from the chaos of the social world. As the age wave continues we elders must put the spiritual central to our lives.   To not do so is like being cut with knives for the messages are everywhere that we are obsolete, of no value—a fiction, a pack of lies! But spiritually we are the highest achievement, essential, transcendent—as high as the skies. The cosmic elder is way beyond cries, since he know his source--it's eternity and heaven he sees with his eyes.

THANATOS: FACING DEATH BRINGS LIFE

It is the presence of death which deepens our appreciation of life and prepares us for harvesting.   The more we embrace mortality as a call to life completion the more anxiety turns to awe, thanksgiving and appreciation. People facing death end their days in zest and joy. All through life they spent energy avoiding reminders of mortality, but this very avoidance saps vitality and hope. All experience of life loses clarity and depth in this denial, which hurts: There's always a free-floating anxiety unsuccessfully drowned out through frenetic activity, entertainment, conquests or obsession with youth. Having de-repressed the fear of death that energy is now released and reclaimed. Wow! Now we feel buoyed up as streams of creative energy courses through the body, mind and nervous system. By facing what usually depressed and terrified we feel lighter, freer and more alive as a shift in attention makes us aware of how precious life is. Then we can accept ourselves, love and lose the anxiety making us grasp at power, wealth and fame to feel confirmed. Then we can truly see the immaturity of youth (often so uncouth). And to think we wanted to be like them or that we actually tried to get their approval!   When we face death even a wonderful humor emerges.   What a relief transcending the boring, mundane, material world of flesh and games and overnight gained-and-lost fames and flames! We come in and go out alone and everyone else is now irrelevant.

FREUD: SEX (STRIVING) OR DEATH (SILENCE)

Freud saw two forces driving the human experience: libido the life instinct and thanatos the death instinct. Life is a ceaseless struggle between these two forces. Libido surges with vitality, seeking pleasure and experience while thanatos longs for silence devoid of all striving and conflict. Libido yearns for sex and creative activity while thanatos drives for death and the cessation of all activity. Freud's view ignores the spiritual for his thanatos is seen as the psyche's bleakest force especially since our culture denies death. It's a serious split since our bodies know about dying and at one point are totally committed to it and yet the culture abhors and avoids it. It deals comfortably with libido expansion and achievement yet panics at contraction, silence and inwardness--the domain of thanatos. Eldering work--the inner journey--embraces and ennobles the death instinct removing its mask and welcoming it's guidance to a much larger life—the comfortable happy existence of mere contemplation and relaxation. Thanatos is the messenger of transcendent love and wisdom—this is God. But how could a culture hating death and aging ever accept the inward life of the saint and mystic? It cannot—it makes it impossible.

DEATH IS THE MYSTIC

Thanatos is synonymous with the ego transcendence and enlightenment portrayed by Hindus.   Yogis break attachment with desire to attain *samahi*--a totally suspended transcendent state of thanatos. Sufis practice *fana*, a blissful state of non-self. Buddhists enter *nirvana*, a desireless state of silence. They all teach there is a natural inborn reflex to seek quiescence as a balance to outgoing energy. Centrifugal complements the centripetal energies. Thanato's inward force brings self-actualization and completion. We are detached from the more indiscriminate social world to extreme selection in relationships and projects attuned to this emerging self: a time to rest and reflect, a time to act and decide, a time to become inspired, a time for creative action and (most importantly)--a time to be very careful in choosing associates (not less careful because you're lonely). Libido and thanatos are bipolar electrical forces with two settings: on/off, life/death, activity/rest. When we are young we make a mark on the world. When we grow old we gradually experience less energy and seek inwardness. The "off" switch is exactly what brings the completion, contemplation and carefully selected actions and friends--all stamped with the seal of growing uniqueness. The OFF is what makes us energetic, attractive, glowing cheekbone-carved older specimens that the younger generation is so grateful for, looks up to and tries to emulate. The ON is what makes us embarrassing caricatures—baby Janes bringing ridicule and rejection—plastic surgery's election, a lost affection, a useless dusty antique collection.

THANATOS   IS   INDIVIDUATION

Thanatos is the urge to individuate--cutting loose everything in the second half of life. Aging people should know they are no longer conquering and expanding but inexorably contracting. For youth, self-preoccupation is a dangerous sin but for an elder it is a necessary duty! Thanatos creates contemplation by limiting libidinal activity. It replaces quantity for quality of experience by insisting we deepen our awareness when we can't expand or conquer any more. But modern drugs like Viagra prevents this natural joyful inwardness--with age libido should shift from sex to mentoring and harvesting and other ways to generate like preserving a legacy through writing and teaching. We are now passing on wisdom, not propagating the species.

THANATOS MEANS COMPLETION, NOT DEATH

CHAMPION GUIDES

Libido is the instinct to begin, while ignoring meaning and wisdom. It's only interested in self's experience--exerting and establishing self in the world. As libido sows seeds, thanatos collects them and brings them as fruits to the harvest. As it's more interested in closure and meaning thanatos is the completing instinct. Only by facing my death could my books come out for thanatos does not always seek physical death but acts as a magnet drawing together and arranging patterns of meaning from our lives. This may mean death or completion of a life's work with decades left to enjoy the bounty coming from it.

When thanatos first appears we panic---exercise madly to compete with youth, redouble our work to prove our worth or have cosmetic surgery--anything but come to terms with thanatos which destroys youth's idols. When mid-life dissatisfaction appears this is thanatos. Having no training for it we mistake the cue-to-completion as a call to death. Not so—the opposite is true: Thanatos marks the appearance of the enlightened self behind the social persona. If we accept it we simply start spending more good time with loved ones, take long walks in nature, play good music and just ponder while looking out the window to the mountain vistas and starlit skies at night. As for me I'm looking forward to old age—it ends the fight, solves the blight, means I'm finally right and higher than a kite.   Baby-boomers unite!

12

From Gabbing and Gorging to

GLAMOROUS AGING

The True Lady is Gentle Worldliness, not Worldly Grossness

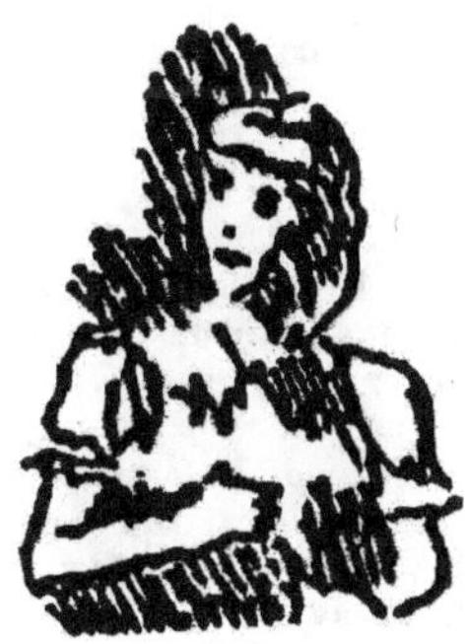

The author has found a brand new life experiencing each moment as a five-year old. I have never been more creative. Each day and hour is flamboyant and lucid with new sights and sounds. All this intensity comes after much difficulty and pain, but a midlife transformation changed all that and now my elder days are packed-in with ecstatic enjoyment. To partake of this bliss one must be strong enough to discount--not take on--the cultural perceptions of aging as an inferior state. We must also know that True Mature Beauty comes from repentance and a contrite heart—then cosmic radiant joy off the chart.

RESURRECTING UNLIVED LIFE

In becoming "adults" we sacrificed parts of self to adapt, but with age these voices clamor for expression. If in retirement we surrender the social image, we can now fish from the deep. Now longings and untapped reservoirs are revealed, for unlived lives are like ringing doorbells we refuse to answer. We stop the ringing by distractions like T.V., but still it screams from the pit: voices of the explorer, the creative child, the student begging for attention, the repressed desire to speak out—to finally have clout. When ignored these betrayed voices go underground, making us seek out the town or just succumb to being unsound. But when in retirement pressures recede and time becomes endlessly unstructured

113

it all comes to the surface starving for attention. Having refused the call of destiny (to choose the inner voice over the outer) now we must complete its call.

If we can't realize unlived life, we should shift awareness to the hidden blessings in the path we took. Now we see our history couldn't have been any other way: For example, I felt shame for food problems but with age began to see it as destiny so I could write books on food, fasting and recovering from compulsion. I could tell the world my war story and how to gain victory. I could develop a diet and routine to banish disordered eating from many lives. So why feel shame? With repentance we gain fame—that's the game as God turns all bad to all good for those letting the self be tamed.

LIFE REVIEW

As elders we re-assemble life in three parts: recontextualizing, forgiving and reclaiming unlived life. In so doing we reshape our experience to see the unique character, charm and meaning of that unique (once-in-a-time) life—despite the weird, ridiculous and "unforgivable" things we did. Most of us received "hot potatoes" from the people shaping our original templates as we inherited judgments, fears and restraints—and these in turn shaped our (often absurd) behavior. In this last life phase we forgive it all while going far deeper--as eldering work examines the template, changes its form and contents and then heals relationship grudges. This inner repair expands self by transcending the petty "I" and re-connecting to nature and God—an expansion bringing real joy and anxiety-relief. Life turns out to be an organic process created by God to enhance us and make us strong, and this global awareness instantly releases cynical depression: For what a joyous experience-- accepting the inevitable rightness of how events unfolded, marveling at the living work of art we've become as the spirit completes us. No matter what, it was right! Wasted decades? No way for these circuitous paths taught us the most. No matter how bleak and painful they created the perfect stew—who we are today, the highest display.

MATURE AGING IS INNER NOT OUTER

When we were young we let groups construct reality and these implants degraded our life from the opulence it could have had when going inward. Now we're better off solo with just a few people with whom we interact. Then the True Self can really alight as we substitute negative cultural stereotypes of aging for positive universal archetypes of elder dignity instead. To get to the joyous universal, give up on the cultural. In universal fairytales age brings richness as meaning continues to expand. With this true maturity, one's inner amplitude (receptivity to the moment) goes deeper so the past collapses and each moment becomes "pithy" with rich meaning. But in the cultural view age is narrowed vision, uselessness, disease and lost meaning. We must never identify ourselves through cultural stereotypes but only via universal archetypes for all cultures are sick to a degree: Only the transcendent is richly relevant (truly mature) human experience.

BELLE AGING: TRUE SEXINESS

Universal aging ("oriental aging") is a positive increase into more meaningful wholes. I call this belle aging, connoting increased beauty and symbolizing "rings-a-bell: speaks with hitting the nail on the head wisdom." We ring-a-bell in the collective unconscious because we are universal archetypes recognizable to all. This is true dignity, having cut away all superfluous elements (culture-race-gender) from the core of the True Self. We are belle-gorgeous, belle-recognized though never seen before. We become the "well-known unknown"--a uniquely one-time-in-history event. The "I" is a symbol of eternity, it's image encrypted on the moon. Belle aging is a sage getting better every day with no envy of youth. Facing death instantly dissolves all the guilts and shames of this temporal life, and freed of these major psyche blocks the elder is "grand": a joy to be around as he helps others through the "shame" and "guilt" from being youthfully outer-directed.

PERSONAL FIREPOWER

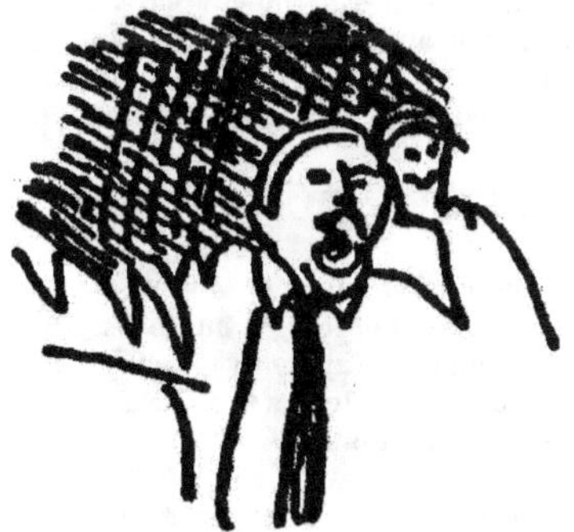

Gorgeous belle aging comes from personal firepower: the explosive vibes that out-dazzle mere anatomy making age irrelevant. Belle aging is pure personality built through years and character--rarified charm, a special presence growing with the years. True "sexiness" has nothing to do with age unless one defines "sexy" in the most stereotyped and boring way—superficially or culturally (a "stud" yet still Elmer Fudd). From the human point of view "sexiness" is a manifestation of personality and character, not of prowess (the way we view lower animals). In and of itself the sex act has little to do with the aura of sexuality a man or woman projects. "Rarified charms" grows as the years write on the face and this is sexiness. Character, personality and aura are hard-won and take time like a fine wine.

AGELESS ALLURE

Take the ageless allure of older movie idols: artists and media heroes seducing the world through the camera. As they grow older their special presence grows, not dims. Each one is a master of his own craft and masterful men are sexy. The central paradox of this charisma is non-dependence on aggressive super-sexuality. What was most winning about Cary Grant was his indifference to such--his muscles never gleamed but his wit sure did: subtlety was his style. He gave "fun" its proper high status and in its pure form, fun is rare. Innocence and subtlety are achievements of time. Having witnessed evil and vulgarity the elder increasingly chooses the purely refined—dry wit, not the gross pits (George Burns not Howard Sterns).

MATURITY IS BEST—IT IS ZEST

"Limitless zest" doesn't wane. Who else but the elder makes "well-being" so subtly attractive? Who else so rarely succumbs to self-pity? These aged humans are never boring but with an infinite capacity for surprise--more growth, more zest. We must grow as ageless children or pay more for remaining "adult." The mature man learns to ceaselessly dare, setting out on new adventures, a picture of the manic energy of youth but with more unvarying excellence, fascination and experimentation with time. Though not eternally young, he is eternally ageless. For him growing older means triumphantly growing into his own skin--no one's ever bored in his presence.   When aged neither vanity nor narcissism dulls his appeal—for he has a right to it as one who relates to spirit (his own and God's).

SUPREME SELF-CONFIDENCE

The older human knows when to talk, when not to and when not to argue with a lush or a louse. As ego recedes he has learned not to fight but to rise above. He tries not to provoke and has learned the fine art of walking away gently. Having transcended cultural stereotypes he can see across race and gender lines. He is of the world—he can truly communicate. The mature elder talks poetry or he doesn't talk.

The mature human possesses supreme self-confidence and this style is the man or woman. Due to panoramic vision he understands love when most complicated, terrifying, hilarious and true and he can love women at their worst: driven, obsessed or threatening. Younger men are always judging stereotypically (old-young, male-female, rich-poor) while older men have seen too many surprises for that. A woman is freer with the elder--as he ages he is more her model for his panoramic vision. The appreciation of True Mature Beauty comes with age as when free of habits that blind he can see eternity. Those who cling to sin to curb anxiety (from aging and stereotypes) succumb to the cultural view of beauty which abandons nature and then oneself—more so with age (hardly a sage). But those who face the reality of nature become their own world's rage.

SEXY OLDER WOMEN

The best thing about the older man is his ability to appreciate the older woman. Belle aging in women shows elegance and sweetness together--the rare lady. The true lady is gentle worldliness not seduction or feminism! The older man sees eternity in her--she represents it all in one ever-changing symbol: always-lovely, well-groomed, long-married, durable, reassuringly stable, home-and-heart devoted, responsible, respectable. She loves everyone in her charge. The man who loves this wife is the most revered and together they make the royal couple. A good example is Joanne Forsythe, an adored wife called "my lady" with reverence--a real sense of adoration for what the wife can do. Her husband constantly provided settings in which the world could see what he saw in her. These older men are the best role models for floundering husbands for due to their long marriages, mellowed-out-maturity and honest affection their strong male presence is expanded. That's all any Queen ever wanted or demanded. A faithful loving husband is the best man ever landed!

SELF-CONFIDENCE TAKES THE PRIZE

These older men could have all fallen victim to the social stereotypes of age but they didn't allow themselves to. Their eternal charm lies in being more themselves as the seasons pass. Their victory over time is to embrace it, for their character and personality increases with age. Self-confidence takes the prize as they disprove all stereotypes about age and lost sex appeal, for self-image grows from years of interacting with others.   Those in the know see older as better—it's the difference between a rat and an Irish Setter.   If men want to be really—authentically—magnetic (i.e. sexy) they should heed the advice of this letter.

OLDER SPIRITS ARE VESSELS: EXEMPLARS

The same holds true in the arts. The older writer is invisible--he is only the vessel through which inspiration comes. He is out of the way yet ever-present: a present from God, an exemplar and yet a paradox whom few know and many may hate. Being above logic, gravity and age he is paralogic---known and controlled only by God who makes no sense to carnal man.   Even he doesn't know why he writes what he does--he just does it without question in each moment and this is the highest possible path. He has given up reasoning and just acts from instinct made more automatic through the years as he releases society. The older human represents eternity and universal (not cultural) truths—this is true wisdom. With time habits dissolve which maintain the ego and thus he is more humble, more loved. What did his ego create when young? By the herd he was shoved.

COALESCENCE
Lucid Life Review

For women aging is particularly hard. Having received their "worth" from childbearing years now past they mourn this loss but then enter a new joyous phase of coalescence--a postmenopausal stage which goes very deep. As everything learned to this point comes together they come to their summit, and this cues the fascinating phase of life-review with intense lucid recall of sights, smells and feelings. Capturing these little gems is many times more interesting than outer entertainment. These little "sparks" of recall may only bore others, for like fasting, prayer or recalling dreams they should be enjoyed alone. If I were to recount these reviews to a friend I would miss the next jewel sparked in consciousness.

CRONES ALONE ARE SHOWN

The crones are postmenopausal single females who are either never taken seriously or burned as witches (too psychic or they use herbs), or they are respected as loving harbingers of new life--health and wealth. Actually the crone is a very smart, creative female who's too busy to abide the intrusion of society. These single eccentrics live longest and are the most productive. Being free, they can give the most to an orphaned and lost world. The crone is the Biblical "eunuch" who is valued by God over the married woman as she loves and takes her orders from God first, while the latter loves spouse and world for the worst.

CEREBETONIA IS GENIUS

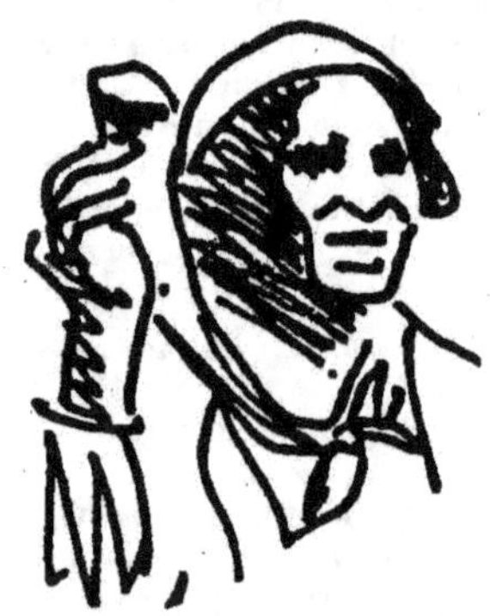

The inability to handle intrusion is a mark of genius and spirituality—it is the very private "cerebrotonic" or savant-autistic (socially separate wizard). She wants only the company of God for none other compares. Every moment is so packed with fascination it's rare the human who could distract from this bliss.   The married take orders from spouse and world, the single enjoy peace with God (all dreams unfurled). Crones and singles enjoy life to the max--the carefree crone is simply someone who no more puts up with puffed-up, prideful, pitiful personalities. That release few can ever know, for it's knowing God instead. It's the absence of being filled with dread, like the past social life she led.

CRONES CAN LOVE—THEY ARE THE DOVE

Crones have a detached capacity to love, uncorrupted by need. Far from lonely they have a great vocation as people instinctively flow in for divine wisdom. In contrast, those fearing age fall into a no-exit trap called avidya (ignorance) by the Hindus: a state of unawareness. fearful contraction and clinging (to people and habits) that denies access to the future where all the glory lies. People who can't look ahead back into the future--moving onward while clinging to what is gone forever. Backing into the future they see only dark failures, broken plans, regrets/resentments, unresolved and ruptured relationships--the emotional "hot-spots" darkening the moment. Shutting off the future leaves nothing but physical decline.

That's not the life of mine. God packs in enjoyment to the very end—that's my tend. I look forward with glee as God increasingly glorifies me.

Resisting the flow of time while editing out signs of mortality leads to depression or a blank psychic field like Alzheimer's Disease. When you reject the truth you are forced to accept a lie--that youth is superior and that aging is sadly inferior. Not so. Paradoxically only conscious aging--accepting death--frees and releases our burden. No more shame, guilt or fear of age, for this very acceptance of death releases true elder beauty and joy. Fear brings wrinkles, the joy of acceptance brings translucency of complexion.   Her laughter brings health and cheer making her a dear as she dries the tear and quiets all fears.

THANATOS IS LIFE—FREE OF STRIFE

The denial of death is a safety factor in youth-"save life at any cost" as threats trigger the fight-flight response of adrenaline pumped through blood. It serves in youth but interferes with eldering when we need only to contemplate, meditate and pray to encounter thanatos without panic. It is in the facing of the terrors of aging and death as part of the spiritual journey that we find courage and wisdom. In confronting death we gain a new orientation in life. Purged of self-concern we awake to the splendors of the moment and little things: flowers, birds, puppies, friends. Released from myopic self-interest and the terror of death we can now serve others. Having been liberated from youth-obsession we become future-oriented, discounting all bad images of "old" by showing the world our zest, joy, service and deep symbolic meaning to everything. Now free of panic the new-found energy pushes open the happy door to "elderhood." We feel much better as the future opens. But to enter this inner sanctuary we must review the past in a healthy light, by recontextualizing failures into successes, releasing resentments and reconnecting to unlived life we sacrificed on the way.

COMING TO TERMS WITH THE PAST

The main task of eldering is to reflect on the wealth of our past experiences. Once life review is set off we have a kaleidoscope of perceptions and revelations like bursts of exhilarated energy. These are lucid sights, sounds and smells that so enrich experience that both life review and enjoying the moment become intense explorations. Eldering is the time of the receptive mode and all the joys of relating to eternity: The phantasmagoria of our own rich history combined with sun-moon-stars. These powerful God-made forces were blocked out in the tunnel-vision of youth's pursuits. It is the flame of accepted mortality which opens this abundant life as we can now see the entire past differently, just as the present--elemental reality of planets and angels--is transformed in our eyes. Our era of conquering and enduring cold love is now over so we can see everything in a brand new light. Now the pain is gone we can see the good in all while staying gentle—a fawn walking tall.

SELF-FORGIVENESS AND SYNCHRONICITY

God says "my thoughts are not your thoughts." We thought we were right but now see we were wrong. We see how much betrayal and treachery were triggered by our own sins. We were blind to our own foibles which were clearly visible to others who reacted accordingly. In youth we jumped to conclusions now re-examined in maturity. When young and vulnerable we saw the world as for or against us--a view reinforced by the hurts and betrayals conspicuous in mind. As age brings breadth these basic views are bashed as we "see" why they turned. We must escape the prison of early conclusions for "the facts were there but my conclusions were wrong."

GOD TURNS ALL-BAD TO ALL-GOOD
It's Jesus' Answer to the hood

Parts of self are still stuck in past pain where stunted experience cries to be healed. We've left home but the wounded child still weeps. Set the prisoners free: It is inner repair which releases us from jail, for unresolved we always fail. The past of strained relationships, sudden trauma and incorrigible irritants forced us into peculiar adaptations. But when we see how these negatives produced the real successes of maturity we can now revisit them saying "yes!" to the pearls the paltry (even perverted) past pains imparted. In all cases no matter what has occurred God turns all-bad to all-good for those who love Him (all bad history becomes blurred). Reviewing the past shows the true gains coming from loss: the higher realm beyond guilt-ridden anxiety reveals the hidden benefits. As mature adults looking back we can do reconstructive surgery on ourselves.   Free of the past and society-- in synchrony with nature--we've become elves as dusty dank memories we've put on the shelves. Instead we go deep inside--the domain into which every spiritual giant delves.

SIN BROUGHT HATE—THEY WERE IRATE

In True Maturity we can see how our own sins removed the hedge protecting us from foes as evil flowed right in. And all these years we blamed everybody else! Or we see how openness to evil elements put us in exile--from ourselves, God and His protections. All we ever had to do was just say NO to flesh and world--our people-tragedies were self-created. Having swallowed that bitter pill we can now take total pleasure in the senses, free of all obsessive-compulsion. True pleasure is non-compulsive!

I was bitter over destiny but now feel grateful to be alive having survived all the challenges of life. Are you riddled with resentment?   Reframe your failures into success by giving testimony for life's severest teachers: list all the past foes and invite them back mentally thanking them for good coming from bad. This alchemy--making gold on aging resentments--converts resentment into gratitude, acceptance and peace. You'll be amazed at how it all fits—how they led to your divine best. The worst in your life, the greatest losses of dignity led to your crest. It is reframing the past and forgiveness which fills you with zest.

FORGIVENESS

It is forgiveness which reformats the templates driving us wild. Using the device of time-stretching we reach back to repair the hurts, broken promises, acts of betrayal and unhealed scars closing our hearts. The grudge keeps us in the dark--there is no creativity, energy or jubilance here.   Forgiveness reveals our own role in the dysfunction and thus we face our shadow--the despised, rejected inner self who trips us up. Self-forgiveness for unconsciously creating the toxic situation unites and then releases the foe as friend for greater life and love. Did your arrogant, stubborn behavior create conflicts? Did the grasping nature of sin trigger cruel hatred in those closest? Daily forgiveness facilitates life harvesting and release--lest they effect the immune system. Reject resentment or fail and die. Forgive, take the throne and prolong your life.

Young beauty is an accident but older beauty is an achievement! If this culture can ever mature we must remove the ageist yoke. It isn't just sexual indecency but the ageist orientation, a youthist coronation: a very low vibration, the making of a degenerate nation. The whole second half of life which should be the most productive so return to our strong beginnings—recover the dignity of our great land: Recover the clan, regain respect for the elders (you can!) and   return to how we began.

Now *because* you've faced death and reframed
your history, you've extended your life accordingly.

Part 2:

EAT THEN DON'T EAT.
ONE MEAL A DAY:

DAILY FASTARIANISM

Fruit or fat is where it's at. The fruit cleans, the fat rebuilds. You need to reverse between both, and fast daily. When you feel fat or in need of a cleanse, go fruit: enjoy sweet like the grape cure or non-sweet fruit like tomatoes, squash, cucumbers, avocados. When you crave more potent foods or strength, switch into fat: enjoy animal fats (fauna) like eggs, dairy, meat or other fats like nut butters. When you hit a glitch, simply switch—but avoid all starch. And fast: life should either be a continuous fast punctuated by tiny potent meals, or eating once or twice a day--you'll love life this way. Being smart is knowing when to switch: for long term fruitarians fail to thrive and despite an initial "high" become fatigued and flat. But eating all fat can turn on you too: feeling fat or blue. After twenty fretful fruitarian years I was happy to see I could safely take fruit vacations--by eating fat. I love life like that! The dual life of diet reversals escapes the problems of both diets while getting the best of both worlds. It's so simple but the hardest for people to grasp: they want one diet, or the other--in such foolish consistencies you will smother, for fruitarian bliss is God's kiss and something you won't want to miss: Without this recurrent cleanse life's amiss, but when you feel constricted or hungry just switch to Swiss. Before we begin I would like to confirm the reversal dieting theory from the standpoint of a medico-paleo-anthropoligist:

Karen: Your reversal dieting theory is true from the viewpoint of medical and paleo-anthropology, for early paleo reversals between fat and fruit combined with fasting is confirmed by every study available. Humans are supposed to be lean and healthy as early man sourced high fat meats/marrow, effortlessly transitioned to ketosis and went without food alternating with fruits. This created a unique trigger that stored and then rapidly reduced body fat when reversing between fat-rich or glucose rich foods. As you point out, primitive man having unstable food supplies had to fast, and fat is the only thing making that tenable along with fruits when readily available. I found your site fascinating confirmation of this early evolution. The combo of nuts and dried fruit is so energy dense you can eat far less to be satisfied. Nutritionists argue you need much more variety for essential nutrients but the body's efficiency with daily fasting offsets this need. Without getting anti-oxidants from a lot of fresh fruits and veggies, by fasting (eating little) immunity goes way up, even minimizing the need for anti-oxidants! You apparently have found a strong and massive readership of people who are ready for it. I commend you in your scholarly work and artistic means of presenting it, for it is rock solid.

Hunter gatherers who live on very high saturated fat/meat diets are also extremely healthy, lean and vital. Humans do very well on paleo foods be they meat or fruits: what westerners do is live on starch combinations--everything and anything with a starch--and these combinations are lethal because they damage beta cells and the brains insulin receptors so they no longer achieve satiety on minimal quantities of food. To get this insulin sensitivity back you have to cut intake dramatically, as you do or eliminate all sweets and starches. I think meat is very good (except hormones may hurt). But raw vegan people are no healthier than anyone else, and suffer from immunity and psychological problems more because of a lack of protein/fat which causes hormonal imbalances . Population growth is destroying our ecosystems and I see the future is grains, grains and more grains: that means more drugs, disease, obesity and lower quality of life, but what can you do The Atkins diet actually accelerates protein loss and they lose substantial lean mass even though they are consuming so much protein... so Atkins can never work long term--only your reversal dieting will work! . Keep to your course for you are completely and totally correct. Dr. L.I. Bennette, University of California.

Author's Note. At 100 lbs. I have no problems with weight due to daily fasting from breakfast-to-breakfast. I include starches now and I'm solid with this weight for life.   But there were many years I had no control and what's written here is how I finally achieved it.

13

FAST FIRST

For Beauty and Synchronicity

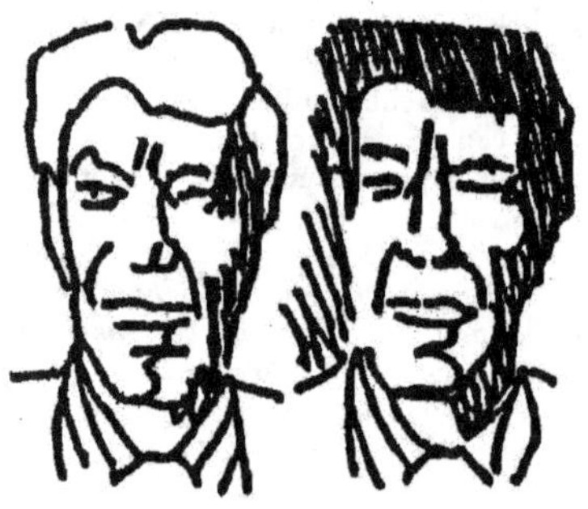

**Fasting has miracle power. The benefits are so great that
once you start doing it you'll be addicted for life.**

REASONS TO FAST

Fasting, the glory of God will manifest and reign in your life. This "day of humiliation" will bring you incredible rewards-"I will increase as you decrease." As you deny your instincts the ego dissolves and then the miracle happens: God takes over and gives you all. This sequence has to occur--it is divine law. To be exalted you must be humbled. To be King you must bow to the floor. To say "I have sinned so I'll fast and pray" precedes your greatest success. Test me on this. You may have reasons to fast, a specific purpose under the direction of God. Not to get attention, not to show off, not to brag to the world what you've given up, no announcement--just something between you and God for power and specific solutions. Fast and tell no one. Fast and be silent. The more humble you are the more power you'll have. If the fast is simply a restriction in each day the rewards are daily and cumulative over time. A daily fastarian (one meal only) is a "mini-faster" and lives in heavenly bliss.

You may be a man or woman of God with real purpose to change society. People are dying for what you have. Through fasting the most ugly can become the most beautiful as all the rough edges blocking success are smoothed out. The way to write, speak or advance a cause is to fast. The silent enemy of your impossible dream is probably not lack of knowledge but not fasting. It's time to prune your life in readiness for a blossoming future. Never grow weary reaching for your impossible dream for God will make a new thing: it will spring forth as He makes rivers in the desert. Fast and it will occur. You must always keep the faith because the world says you won't make it: "it's been too long...you're over the hill...you're too old." Fast and this will all be false. Shun the cold, go for the gold. Just finish your work--and do it in bold.

Fasting is healthy.   It brings power—dynamite, supernatural power to get revelation, protection, spiritual gifts and deliverance from addiction. "Let the oppressed go free" as it breaks every yoke to be the genius of the family tree in pursuit of the highest calling, the jubilee. Fast for guidance when you don't know what to do. Fast for healing no matter what disease. Fast for miracles when you need to know something unknowable in the natural. Fast for excellence: We're surrounded by mediocrity--don't succumb and become part of it- -just fast and reign over it. Rise up to exemplarship. Fast and the supernatural kicks in. If you want freedom from controllers, fast. If you want freedom from your bad habits, fast. God wants to release you from all these yokes, so fast! When you don't know what to do, God will show you what to do. Nothing is impossible--so just fast and the miracle arrives. Don't limit God by your low-minded natural thinking. He rules only by the supernatural-- the impossible. Fast to overcome evil: just be patient while they get theirs: "I will not bow down" but I will fast.

Fast first to be lighter, purer, wiser and to have power in public. God's beauty will be in and all around you. Step into a much higher reality--first in spending time with God then spinning out to each abundant moment. You'll find yourself in a whole new world, another reality of beauty and profound self-confidence. It's the key to this higher world. You'll be amazed at the diseases healed (even your hair is curled). Your competitors will pale as powerless in your perception. It's the way to win, to overcome, to step up to the plate, to strut your stuff fast forward, to end all sin.

Do you realize how just one slight change can transform your whole life suddenly? This was my realization when I began to eat one predawn then spend heavenly days with God in contemplation and then a wonderful cozy sleep. There was a sudden transfiguration and a wonderful dis-fattening. I hate blubber on the frame and my sudden slimness brought great relief. As the fat came off so did the evil memories, the shameful things in life that hold us down until we die. They were gone--they died through diet. It was as if my whole life was waiting for just this switch. Everything changes: one's life, looks, outlook and overcoming power in a cruel world.

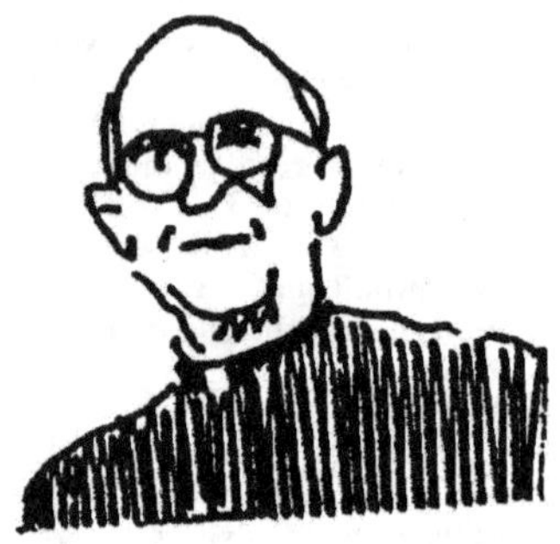

All Religions Use Fasting!

Though it should be the opposite, after forty we're all at a disadvantage in this world. Fasting levels the playing field as now you become your best and most energetic all day. If you eat higher paleo you'll be heavenly satisfied though empty--and this emptiness will act as a magnet to your seed symbol: the way you're supposed to look in your highest intelligence and wit. It can mean the difference between complete success and humiliating failure. It was for me as digesting anything became counter-productive to all that I wanted to do. I tried Atkins--three squares a day--but the fat wouldn't come off nor the creative take-off. I finally saw God was urging me to fast after a little fruit and fat and then it all came off— just like that.

THE KEY IS FASTING: A PRIVILEGE

I love to fast and I've learned to thank God for the privilege. This attitude always removes the pain or weakness. If it's a 60-hour weekend fast I think of how good I'll feel when its over and just enjoy the experience as the two days speed by. If I'm fasting it's a good excuse to sleep and really relax. Fasting is a wonderful vacation like being on an all-expenses-paid holiday. You'll find you're in a fairyland where miracles never cease.

When you feel fat, forget dieting and just do things the old-fashioned way: fast. It will give you unimaginable self-esteem and confidence. It's a test of the true warrior in you, the one who is strong enough to deny an impulse in respect to a principal. The rest of us just make promises only to break them when feelings change. Not you, who will be rewarded with great character for taking the plunge and finishing it. It really separates you from weaklings controlled by desire. You'll be amazed at how habits and memories fall away. I used to go on fruit fasts but now find no food is the best for character-building. Just eat the sun and live on God.

When you do eat you'll do best on higher paleo—fruit and fat as you go back to prehistoric roots. After twenty years of fruit-only and the degeneration which came from a fat-free diet

I existed solely on one daily fat meal for one year and it brought total rejuvenation. It is the combination of the fat, fruit and the fast that worked. I wanted championship and that is achieved through proper diet combined with daily fasting--the highest art of the ages that performs miracles and eradicates evils that would never leave any other way. I can't believe what a change it's made in my life.   From dreary, depressed mornings when I would often take a nap to whirlwind mornings of activity joy and optimism. It is rather unbelievable and a wonderful midlife development when we really need a boost. Fasting was the key unlocking mysteries and powers surpassing any previous era of my life. The whole point to bring out one's talents is routine, routine, routine! Become a methodist---method is the key-lock to success. Focus by eliminating all non-essentials including food. Let your new slogan be: avoid non-essentiality.   No one really needs more than one meal a day so now open yourself to new adventures.

Routine being the essence of assured success soon, what are the best ways of doing things? It will all be made clear through your daily fasts. As all loose ends come together everything will look different. The past is caught in new webs, while shame and guilt disappear. It was all just dead memory stored in fat: holistic images becoming more distorted with each recall. As you dis-fatten you'll become a totally new person with new associates and a real life. What a relief as you now have fond memories of the past which is seen in the opposite way. People won't recognize you with the transformation.

I had many resentments and memories causing anxiety. All this dissolved along with the "false body" built with wrong foods or constant eating. It's just like a dusty mirror being cleaned off. This didn't happen with fruitarianism as fat deficiency combined with too much sugar caused depression and continuously elevated insulin resulting in emotional instability and "state-dependent memory". The bad emotional state we are in determines the bad events we remember! With the higher paleo diet you'll feel so good and even, so memory will become "kind" as proper food cleanses the mind. Your thoughts will stay immersed in the beautiful here-and-now and you'll have only fond memories of the past. Fasting achieves this better than fruit because nitrogen and solar radiation are the highest nutrients when free of sugar--which can kill the mood and change the emotional state. The body re-adapts to grasp these higher God-creations of sun and air when not given grosser foods. Fasting is a lost art and as the Bible says "fast and pray daily": eating one meal a day is doing just that as we enter a brand new life based on maximum digestion and assimilation of food, total creative power, favor with man, attraction of good elements and repulsion of bad. You're protected in this state--a blissful state you step into. Once there you'll never want to come back.

FRUGAL FRUITARIANISM
WITH FAT, THEN FAST

Maximum Meal Map Sample
a.m.: Fruit or smoothie
Cheese Omelet or Greek Red Salad
Fast to next day.

Let's get started on what to eat between your fastings so sweet. Enjoy some raisins and figs when first hungry in the morning—raisins are the grapecure for cancer. These black fruits filled with iron and magnesium for energy and cleansing pull poisons from the bloodstream. For the main meal make doughless pizza by melting cheese with nuts and garlic powder or make tomavo with avocado, tomato and lemon juice in the blender. Add peppers cilantro and garlic for guacamole. If you want a salad make Red Salad by slicing red peppers, tomatoes, avocados and perhaps some leaves with lemon juice and olive oil. These non-sweet red fruits are incredibly cleansing and nutritious without spiking insulin. Add some cheese for Greek Red Salad. Satisfied? Now fast to the next day or if hungry have some raisins and nuts at night. No diet is simpler but will give you the largest life filled with light (see recipes www.karenkellock.com).

LIGHT PALEO LUNCH

Sugar and starch are killers and put the body in fat storage mode. But fat evokes the fat-burning mode characterized by highest energy and appetite suppression (ketosis).   I have happily seen the super-obese slim down on this regimen and experience no toxic cleansing effects save a mild fatigue.   Fats provide enough density to slow cleansing and the less aggressive action makes this period very happy—our moods becoming even for once. Then the afternoon fast takes off from this blissful lunch elevation   and the result is a beautiful productive day—more so each day as one becomes slim, trim and youthful-looking--the result of fruit-cleansing and fat-nourishing moistening. Fat and fruit is the HQ (highest quality) food so you require very little for highest energy and appetite-suppression for the day. These facts are obvious as disordered metabolisms clear up without any deficiencies whatsoever. I also love the colon-happy efficiency and regularity that the fat and fiber in the fats like avocado or cheese with nuts create. Throughout the chapters below you'll see the necessity of fauna-fat (animal protein) like cheese--when combined with the purifying action of fruit and the fast the results are amazing and cumulative.

FOOD AND MOOD

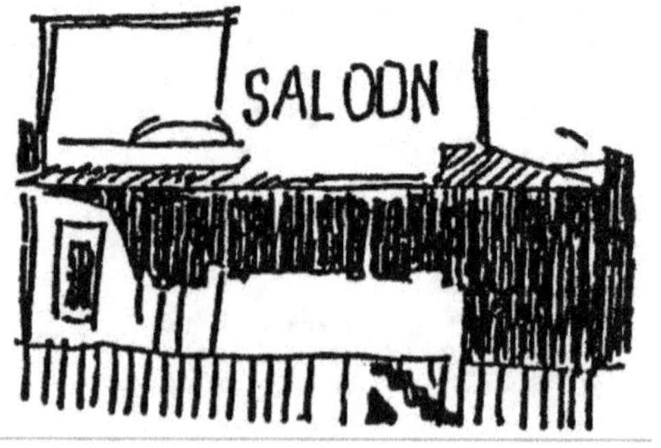

You don't have to resent the past or mistrust all people because of early pain. These are all distorted implants made worse as we get older. Having eaten at those events we accumulated more "layers" of false body (made by false foods) and the result was growing "widening" misperceptions. These early templates get progressively worse until in midlife we'd better dissolve the template or die. The patterns which "define" us worsen as they combine with wrong eating, leading to physical build-up. Memories are stored in tissues and in fixed patterns--these must be dissolved for a clean slate in the psychology of food addiction: One eats to erase the past which continues to inflame when hunger sets in again.

Break this block. Start your fast with a mental diet--consciously eliminate all bad mental habits: negative thinking or the nonessential thoughts which get worse through mutual reinforcement. They make you want to eat to dissolve their intensity--a distraction from pain--but eating never works despite the illusion that it does. As these "layers" unpeel back to the root you'll experience the exact same memories simultaneous with that era. You must re-experience the whole movie as it rewinds and the result will be bliss—when the fog lifts you'll be left standing there: a beautiful ageless and happy child of God as you were at the beginning. The champion's goal is to become childlike once more—that indicates he's almost to shore and the past is out the door. Proper diet and fasting will clean him to the core, and it won't be a chore as his reality becomes fascination galore.

CLEAN THE VEINS THROUGH FAT

You must clean your veins (and your memory) through fat. As it elevates glucagons and the body goes into fat-burning mode carb-addiction and the memories it feeds will be gone. As long as you stick to starchy carbs like grains you'll be storing fat, making more memories to mess the machine up with mismanaged eating. Switch to fat, fruit and fasting and you'll blow out these nasty circuits instead. Nothing eradicates memories more than just maintaining an even mood through the correct diet—not eating that which sits like lead (bread).   Carbs will leave you tired depressed and craving as you relapse into the past instead.

FRUIT BINGING IS NOT PURITY

Take note of all the changes with insulin from starch and sugar: head-aches, insomnia, bloat and distention, water retention, rashes and welts, dryness, irritability, depression, indigestion, gastritis, uncontrolled anger, constipation, cravings, fatigue, sleepiness, stupor, breathlessness, constriction, closing up arteries, fat storage, the making of cholesterol stupor and dizziness. This all reminds me of the last time I ate bread and jam, but in a person with sugar disorder even fruit causes these maladies. Because it makes man himself, fat-fasting (with the cessation of sugar and starch) is the thing which is spiritual, not the produce and grains which "seem" so "Godly". The fruit (higher paleo) diet is not austere but makes you feel good with none of these problems, not a tear.

As a fruitarian I was seeking "purity" through food while eating fruit all day. That's not the point--we don't gain from eating but from fasting. We "break out" of yokes by not-eating, by stopping the motion--the mindless repetition. Eating takes us nowhere while fasting takes us everywhere. Begin mind-traveling. Let your thoughts spin out to outer space as every day is new, fascinating, adventurous and gay. Create your own reality in your own environment and God will be with you.

OP-TRUTH: OPTIMISTIC FASTING

Give up the carnal in pursuit of the spiritual. Spending time with God is the answer and fasting is a wonderful way to do that. You'll go beyond the obvious--which makes you oblivious--and see wonderful deeper meanings to things, new avenues never seen before. Many if not all things will be seen in the opposite way. Remember our slogan "OP-TRUTH": the opposite to what people think, what circumstances (mere appearances) indicate or what you feel may be the truth. When things seem boring and empty it may be that everything is happening underground, about to burst into wonderful success! When the world seems against you, it may precede your meeting the love of your life. "OP-TRUTH" gives relief from the uncouth, a new way to sleuth.

Most importantly God's ways and thoughts are higher than man's--they are not just different they are opposite. Fast, suspend your brain and illuminate. Fast and wait on God--something good's about to happen. Prepare for visitation, your promised rewards. You're here for a reason—your work is the Lords. The more you fast in optimism the more you'll love doing it and thank God for the privilege of ascension to this greatest spiritual reality. Use this key to victory and experience such great bounty every single day of your long life: the Daily Fastarian is King. Surrounded by gluttons fasting makes our heart sing--with this divine device we conquer everything.

HOLY DAILY FASTARIANISM

Fasting has so changed my life I decided to devote a chapter on each type of daily fast. You'll be so proud and self-confident when you see the edge you'll now have in society. Congratulations! You've chosen the right book and today you're going to see it. You don't need therapists and books on psychology--just the key to your own inner realm where all the answers lie. The fast is as high as the sky. Are you angry about something your anger can't change? Fast at it—gone is your cry. It'll all dissolve--those things so significant today are as vapor tomorrow. When filled with fat we make mountains out of molehills while fasting brings joy and thrills.

HAPPY HOLY FAT-FASTING

Besides fasting we're going to dissolve fat by eating fat. Dietary fat releases lipid mobilizers--fat mobilization substance that burns the fat off the body. It takes fat to fight fat but only the most independent thinkers will be able to hold on to that point. We have been so brainwashed against the word "fat" while remaining naïve about metabolic truths which oppose herd dogma--i.e. the current fat phobia. We even hear physicians spouting the anti-fat party line, another op-truth. It takes a very strong mind to oppose the masses and their doctors on this issue as the "anti-fat" campaign seems a self-evident truth.   But I will demonstrate that fruit-fat like avocado is not enough. You must also take fauna—cheese, eggs or fish to experience the total appetite suppression for the fasting day, and to keep your engine humming at its highest after the "fruit honeymoon" is over. Pure fruit or vegan diets work well at first but in the long term they become a curse.

There are only three macronutrients or foods that we eat: fat, protein and carb. Fat and protein usually go together so when people delete fat they must substitute with carb starches--laying on fat more than ever. Starch and sugar raises insulin which cues the body to store everything as fat. Raise insulin from carbs and you'll be wearing everything you eat. Eat more fat and raise the opposing hormone glucagons which burns it all instead. You'll get thin through fat-fasting as fat--when free of carbs--puts you in ketosis, the fat-burning mode. After eating your fatty meal wait for appetite suppression to take over. It may not occur for a few minutes but when it does you'll feel full.

IT TAKES FAT TO FIGHT FAT

Look around--everyone's fat. why? Because they've deleted fat and substituted carb. Very fat people continue to delete fat and replace it with more carbs, never putting things together. They cannot imagine it could be the opposite to what they think. Glucagons burns fat. View the difference between the two hormones and you can see how crucial it is to eat fat:

INSULIN.: Insulin lowers blood sugar, shifts the body into fat-storage mode, converts glucose and protein to fat stored on the body, converts all dietary fat to storage, removes fat from the blood and puts it in more fat cells, increases the body's production of cholesterol, makes the kidneys retain water, stimulates growth of arterial cells (closing the arteries) and stimulates the use of glucose--not our own fat--for energy.

GLUCAGONS: Glucagons elevated from fat does the opposite: it raises low blood sugar, shifts the body into burning mode, converts protein and fat to glucose for energy, converts dietary fats to ketones for the highest energy, releases fat from the fat cells for energy, decreases the body's production of cholesterol, makes the kidneys release all water and salt (streamlining the body) and stimulates the use of your own fat for energy--the highest energy possible.

LOWCARB DIETS

So now the world is going lowcarb all the way. That is an over-reaction I say—and you will pay. Deleting fruit is not the answer for it is the master cleanser and highest vibration. A diet of mainly animal products is too toxic—how about some fruit and a little cheese--the European way? Forget calories and carbs altogether for as long as you've deleted starchy refined carbs like rice, beans, pasta and bread you'll lose weight and then enjoy all the starches you want in your ONE MEAL. For now just stick to frugal fruit, non-sweet salads, fats through avocado-nuts-cheese in the "food time" preceding your daily fast—and never count calories and carbs again. Now just relax into your new carefree (fail-free) life for the main point is the daily fast. That will create your new life of beauty, the Godly design into which you've been cast.

THIN IS FUN

The thinner I am the more creative. That's a fact I sensed intuitively as a teen-ager. Birdlike engines prove Einstein's point that less is more as most creative energy comes in least mass. Being thin brings synaptic clarity: perfect conductivity, a continuous mood elevation and freedom from past-fact-stored-in-fat. Fasting dissolves swine consciousness as we become truly noble human beings. Eating-thrills create ignobility, so go from the crass and carnal to the class--supreme class of the superior human being made pure through self-denial and discipline. You'll soon say: "The fast is the feast. All my problems have ceased."

WITTY INVENTIONS

Witty inventions are the way to prosperity--they are the gifts to the world through us. They don't come from logic but just dawn on us when receptive, and fasting sets the stage. Fasting has been the key from the beginning as central to all religions. It opens man to himself and God--to all the answers he'll ever need. Accordingly fasting and correct diet is the most important subject for a book: fat-fasting. As you begin doing both you will see why. Fast--to dissolve ego and the false body--to get to the power of the universe. Fast--for you must have the wisdom of God to invent and then to stay on top. Fat-fast--so the properly fat-nourished brain will illuminate when you are fasting. Then you'll go directly into your own inner journey, away from the maddening crowd and all its recent hits. Inside no one can steal your joy--you're now on top, no more the wet mop.

Whenever you feel "sick" with low self-esteem you will know you've been around the herd of gainsayers--the majority view which actively and jealously resists all your views. Association with the socially hypnotized hurts.   It takes your right out of the receptive joyous mode into tunnel-vision--the addictive past eating you alive. The result? Desire for the food-fix. When you eat at slights nonverbal or otherwise your life becomes a series of ups and downs. The food addict becomes a severe disappointment to friends, family and especially spouse. Do you eat more when hurt? You must fast to overcome, not lay down and be weak (eat) to be hit again—your sin. They're looking to find fault for your gifts bring envy and prejudice. You must fast and all these obstructions shall be overcome—that's this whole book in sum.

FASTING AND THE SEVEN NEEDS OF MAN

Fasting fulfills the seven needs of man so beautifully and quickly. They are: (1) Love. No matter what our sordid history regarding love, fasting puts us in a much higher state where we are love and we attract it all around. It's a way to win favor with God and man. (2) Pleasure. "In his presence is fullness of pleasure and joy." We ascend to a higher state above our old fears, hatreds, jealousies, guilts and shames. These all dissolve in the fasting state of beauty, greatness and achievement. (3) Beauty. We should want to be beautiful to look at.

Fast and the Lord changes the countenance. (4) Greatness and success. Have you always felt you were destined for something great? This will bring it to light. Just fast and say what Moses said: "show me your glory." (5) Freedom to show our emotions. Your self-expression will be given power, refinement and artistry. Have some class: show your emotions for the fasting genius is always in good taste and all will relate. (6) Joy: you shall have it--the sense of continual accomplishment will put you in constant joy unspeakable. (7) Desire to be recognized and remembered after death. We all have a destiny and purpose. Fasting will illuminate this for you and whatever you wish and hope for--your destiny--will be far greater. The greater the destiny the more important the fast. You'll never want to be seen in a non-fasting state in public again. Fast to "behold His glory and be in His presence all the days of my life." This fasting glory is the atmosphere of heaven come down to earth.

DAILY FASTING IS THE KEY TO
AGELESSNESS AND JUST A KID AT 90

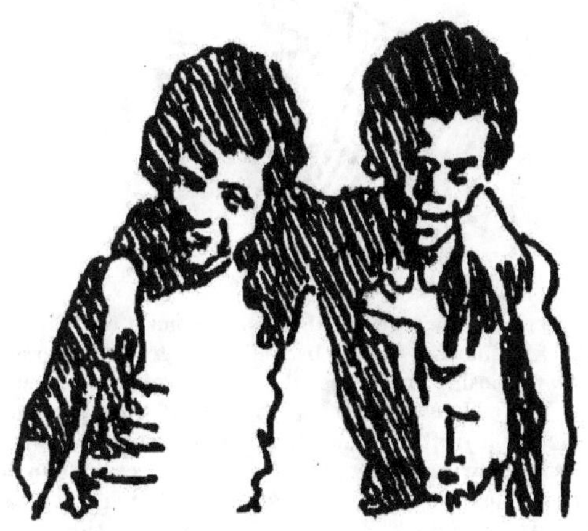

14

REVERSAL DIETING

The <u>Two</u> Sciences of Metabolism
Must be Understood Before we
Proceed with Fun Fabulous Fasting

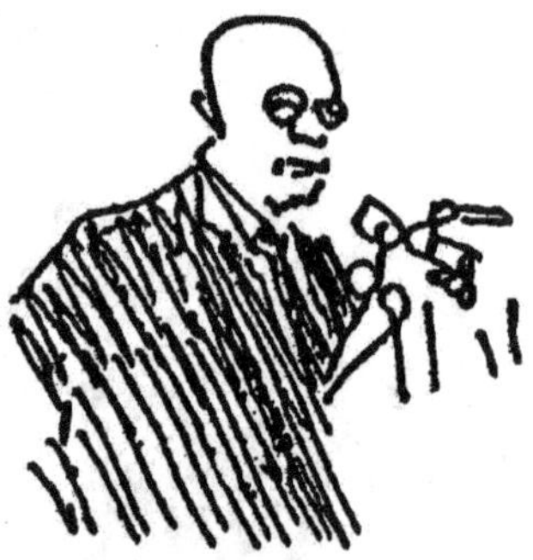

The answer to our miseries is the reversal of diets. It's not a controversy between fruit or fat (between Ehret or Atkins) but rather becoming a very wise person because of your knowledge of both. Not choosing one or the other but reversing constantly to fit the needs which I will describe. You will know when to go fruitarian, when to go lowcarb and when to fast. When I regressed as a fruitarian and suddenly switched to no-carb for one year to revive my protein and fat-deprived system that was the perfect thing to do. I was extremely energetic and happy on a no-carb and fasting diet of just one daily meal of cheese omelet. But then just as suddenly the body said "I want fruit" and the only thing that worked best was now the grapecure and fat in the form of raisins and cheese--but no eggs. Now I'm happy with raisins or figs when hungry and later cheese and nuts—and the rest of the time light lemon aid. The fast is the point so about all those meals don't get out of joint. Just enjoy your fasting life which God will anoint.

REVERSALS ARE THE POINT

Everyone's perfect diet is endlessly mutable while staying within the general fat-fruit-fastarian matrix.   The fruitarian theory says fruit is such a beautifier but yet the elevated insulin brings bloat and bad skin when at a certain stage—when the protein deprivation overrides any benefit from the fruit. It's all a matter of where you're at. I chose to be lacto-nut-fruitarian as home base but will eat vegetables, salads and fish if I ever go to restaurants. After so much fruitarian isolation what a relief to feel a part of the world again—to be able to eat most of what my hostess serves yet to still have the "fruitarian highness"–the reality I so crave. I'm talking about fruit and fasting afternoons while maintaining maximum energy because you are properly fat-fed.

The most important answer is the fast. The superior man is a fat-frugivorous fastarian. If you eat your main meal at noon then like the Buddhist monk focus freely on your fast in contemplation, study, a nap, exercise, leisure. You must know you are fasting to pat yourself on the back. You ate, now you're fasting. It's no big thing to eat at noon and then not eat again until the next morning but it's a full twenty-hour fast. You're a faster and gaining all the benefits thereof. Don't let anyone criticize because it's not thirty days. The daily faster makes it a life routine and has no need for long and painful fasting regimens. Eating the right food for man once a day makes you King and Queen for that day. Be smart: reverse in between these two poles but eat vegetables and leaves on occasion—when you eat at high-class restaurants as a major VIP!

DETOX OR SLIMMING-REBUILDING MATRIX

Here are the two different sciences of metabolism: one propounded by Ehret (detox matrix) and one by Atkins (fatburning-rebuilding matrix). By way of illustration I will describe the Grapecure for cancer first.

GRAPECURE
Detox Matrix

Ehret's detox matrix goes like this: the human body is an elastic pipes-and-tubes system of 62,000 miles of fine capillary with an inner tissue system that resembles a sponge. Anything but fruits and green vegetables creates mucus which nature adapts to by storing in the tissue system. The average person is carrying around twenty pounds or more of morbid matter-- debris stored from head to toe. It is mucus, feces, pus, poison deposits, morbid watery flesh and decomposing tissue. This awful mess putrefies into "disease." The specific 4000 disease- names refer only to the specific point of encumbrance. "Modern man is a walking cesspool" said Ehret as the entire pipe system is encrusted. Worse, 70% of autopsies show decades-old feces and worms. This mess becomes cancer as well as all other diseases. So heal by cleaning out the impacted debris (The Debris Theory of Disease). Here's one type of fruit-fasting which is especially perfect for cancer-cleaning:

GRAPECURE FOR CANCER BUILDUP

The Grapecure is in three stages: 1. complete dissolving of the encumbrance. 2. complete elimination of poison. 3. complete rebuilding of new tissue. This thorough regeneration is what marks the grape. Cancer cannot be cured through fasting since it checks the growth but is again strengthened when food is re-ingested. The grape eliminates cancer curing entirely. It is the "Queen of the Fruits" with the highest dissolving action and the most complete nutrient. Man can enjoy a long vacation on the grape as the amino acids become proteins plus all needed nutrients. All abnormal growths and tumors are dissolved by this powerful chemical reaction. The cure is mentioned in the Bible as a divinely simple gift to suffering humanity. Often used as a last resort the grapecure shows complete recoveries despite hours to live. The patient must have faith, a strong desire to live and the network must encourage the healing process.

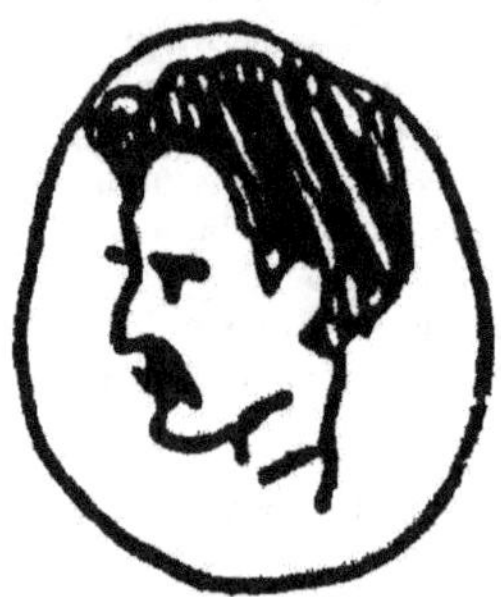

Stage One: Dissolving encumbrance. This is grape-only (juice grapes or raisins) every two hours from 8 a.m. to 8 p.m.. This stage takes 7-10 days and it is here that painful symptoms may occur. The patient should take joy in these points of pain since it indicates that cleansing is occurring. Until the encumbrance is dissolved the real relief does not begin and the grape does not stop until all is eliminated. The now-stirred-up poisons must come out lest they auto-intoxicate the blood again so one to two enemas must be given daily if no bowel movements occur.

Stage Two: Elimination of Poison. Grapes will be combined with other fruits but not at same meal: grapes (8 a.m.) fruit (10a.m.) etc. Having eliminated the biggest chunks, deep cellular cleansing now begins. Old pus, poisons, prescriptions and foods from puberty release from cells into the blood. Cell-cleansing is the most intense part of the cure.

Stage three: Rebuilding of New Tissue. A complete regeneration of all organs will now occur. The salt balance is restored with tomato, red bell pepper, cucumber, lemon and olive. This "red salad" at noon is preceded with juicy fruit in the morning and prunes or raisins at night. Daily elimination should now work perfectly. The worst is over as each day shows more beauty and health. The ratty cellulite-coarseness and wrinkles of the skin (from debris storage) becomes baby-fine moist smoothness as debris is broken up and dispersed. Perfection is achieved!

The most common mistake of the medical profession: The patient cannot eat (injurious fasting) followed by eating solid foods (for "nourishment"). This process is followed by an eruption of the cancer which was arrested through fasting but then gathers stronger hold with eating. The only answer is the grape regimen.

LOW-CARB DIETING

CHAMPION GUIDES

Slimming-Rebuilding Matrix

A high percentage of people in the West have so over-indulged in sweets and starch that they have developed hyperinsulinism. When we eat carb the body secretes insulin to store the glucose until a time it is needed--we store fat. In over-starched and -sugared cultures the insulin receptors are overworked and so more and more insulin is secreted each time. Soon everything we eat is stored as fat. Obesity is everywhere and 70% of Americans have hyperinsulinism. One cure: limit carbs drastically for once the condition has occurred it only gets worse and no diet will work without severe carb-restriction. We are speaking of refined carbs particularly, while fructose is actually cleansing without elevating insulin if eaten frugally. (Note: After his initial weight loss Atkins said he ate 80 carbs a day of fruit and stayed thin.)

The degenerative diseases associated with hyperinsulinism are coronary heart disease, arteriolosclerosis, diabetes and hypertension. For someone who overindulged in sweets and starch early in life the insulin receptors are so worn out that just one touch of glucose sends insulin pouring forth dropping blood sugar levels low (fatigue) while storing fat and water. Sludgy, stodgy and sullen we become tired, irritable and hungry!

I COULD FEEL IT HAPPENING...

Insulin constricts: all the airways and vessels squeeze in as insulin acts as a vasoconstrictor. As it holds water this means hypertension as everything closes down. I felt as though I was suffocating as all the airways closed in. Look at the difference between the two states: Insulin suppresses the immune system, increases inflammation and pain, decreases oxygen flow, decreases endurance, causes platelet aggregation (growth of artery cells thus constricting blood vessels) and proliferates rogue cells (this is cancer). The result is breathlessness, headache, cramps, swelling and rashes. It is not FAT which brings on heart attacks but carb! In the absence of carbs, fat is totally harmless!

Glucagons on the other hand brings a vasodilation (opens up), enhancing immunity, decreasing pain and inflammation, increases oxygen flow, increases endurance, prevents platelet aggregation, dilates airways and decreases cell-proliferation (cancer). Cancer, heart disease, diabetes and arteriosclerosis is sugar/starch-based--having nothing to do with dietary fat.

KETOSIS!
Appetite Suppression

Under glucagon's stimulation the body burns fat rather than stores it. When the body lives off of fat it is the glorious state called ketosis. Ketones are the energy the brain and heart prefer to live on. Contrary to cultural phobias surrounding dietary fat it is not the problem. The pervasive fat-phobia is simply a knee-jerk reaction to the word "fat" with no attention to the metabolic processes that follow the ingestion of fat (without carbs) versus eating carbs. Glucagons--from lowcarb and high fat is the hormone of fat burning and fatty tissue breakdown, reversing the storage processes put in motion by insulin. The puffiness of water retention is present with insulin yet instantly releases with glucagons. We need fat to fight fat. The ketogenic diet releases fat mobilizers--secretions released into the bloodstream to dispense and burn fat. A study by Benoit showed that if eating pure fat and no carbs these lipid mobilizers were released and the subjects lost their fat stores twice as fast as when they fasted. When he put patients on a "fat-fast" with small bits of fat incrementally through the day the weight-loss outdid the total fast by 88% of loss of body fat.

The other diet-happy thing about fat is that it is a complete appetite-suppressant. When we are in Ketosis--the condition of burning rather than storing fat--we lose all appetite while having more energy. We are fat-burning machines living happily on our own fat, ecstatic for life with no cravings for sweets or any other "comfort" food. After two days all cravings leave and we are totally satisfied. I am amazed how just a piece of cheese for breakfast deletes hunger for the day so I can forget food and just enjoy the ray.

FAT PHOBIA IS A CULTURAL HYPNOTIC

The prevalent panic over dietary fat is a cultural hypnotic. It makes no sense scientifically once one knows the metabolic processes that follow the eating of fat vs. carb. We should be a lot more afraid of being fat but not at all afraid of dietary fat when eating without carbs.

Someone may start on this high-fat/low carb diet and be enormously happy with it, only to be talked out of it by friends and associates! Can't anyone think independently anymore? The fat-phobia is the biggest example of social hypnotism I can think of. If one eliminates all fat from the diet he has to eat something so the only thing left is starchy-sugary. It is very common with vegetarians to substitute over-starch for the deletion of meat.   Many vegetarians are still fat. The consequences of eliminating fat and then gorging on starch and sweet are devastating--never have we had such an obese nation of adults and children.

15

FASTING MIRACLES

Just Start and Life Fits Amazing New Winning Pattern

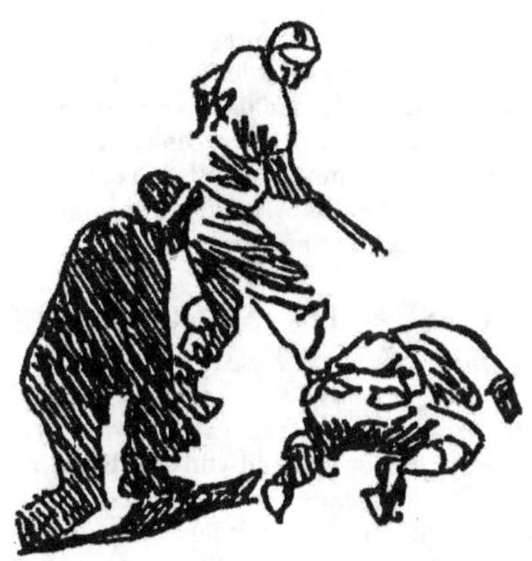

It's a cruel world and life gets harder as we age, right? It doesn't have to be. The only way out of a future of despair in an ageist society is to live in a brand new world of fasting miracles. Just drastically change your life, starting today. Then the results will also be drastic: your metamorphosis will be unbelievable and soon, so get ready and look ahead. Be afraid to eat, for it will destroy the beauty of life and yourself, smudging the vision of God inside. Eat wrong and you'll fall from luminous translucency of skin and feature to dingy white and fuzzy, nondescript and indistinct features--not being sharply defined and looking very ordinary. Which would you choose? Your thought life will be just as disparate from magically great and optimistic to boringly ordinary and cynical.

The faster lives in a separate reality of magic castles and endless possibilities. It's all his, for fasting is all. You can now throw away your psychology books and sessions--they're of no value compared to the profoundly deep inner insights about to occur. Fasting, your True Self sees all through direct access to God, the designer of the unique blueprint you're about to display. Fast to explore the millions of mansions in your soul. You'll never be bored or lonely again.

When you feel the walls closing in, when you feel your heart breaking, when you have no where else to turn, go to your last resort--the fast will work every time. In the twinkling of an eye the mere decision to fast will make mountains into molehills as it changes your pauper status to kingship. It will change your NO--"it cannot be done" to YES-"it 's all mine." This trump card of last resort usually begins with tremendous heart pain---either from people or a sense that life is passing you by. I speak to the baby boomers--many of you sit in panic, feeling obsolete. Not true. Fasting will change the tune--then you will see as you move into all you're meant to be. You know that terror inside that can lead to suicide? Change the tide as the fast releases your infinite talents inside. Let the terror of obsolescence be a call to fast for your mere decision releases positive healing forces (PHF) that will start the Big Change that will astound you. You're not over the hill--you're just beginning, for with the fast the impossible can be done, and all in fun.

Become firm--not infirm and weak. The minute you do you'll feel the growing power that will change your life. I'm not asking you for a long fast but just the fasting consciousness of one mini-fast each day. Just by skipping one meal you can experience the miraculous new life. Why isn't this a world rage? Because it's a Dionysian generation who just wants the pleasure of eating irrespective of the damning results. People get mad at the word "fast" not realizing the miracle that occurs. That is what keeps it bound like a secret society. That secret is owned only by a few, now including you.

FROM SIN TO SYNCHRONICITY
Bipolar Fast vs. Feast consciousness

There are two sides of the brain and two separate nervous system. That is two sides of reality--the good and the bad. The boring dead-end and the miracle of infinite possibilities. It's the difference between sin or grating with the universe, and synchronicity where everything fits together in one miracle after another. Let's compare the two states.

When in the eating state the energy is pulled from the brain to the gut and "miracle consciousness" is lost. You're now in dense dys-synchrony: tunnel-vision and diligence ending in frustration. In the fasting state the energy stays high in the brain and now you're clear: hello magic synchronicity. You're now totally receptive to the moment where past and future unite, pithy with new excitements and joys, new thoughts and fascinating avenues of discovery—a much higher vibration.

Your perception of the world can regress to hell through food—it suddenly seems like a prison to be avoided. Just for the temporary pleasure of eating, energy is blocked as the system closes down through fear. With the energy in the gut the world may seem chaotic, disordered, bland and boring. In the fasting state the world becomes your arena of pleasure and learning--it seems friendly and fascinating as you open up through love and creative energy flow.

Your placement in the world is also bipolar: in the addicted tunnel-vision state we feel separate, isolated or stilted. We fake "social consciousness" from fear of rejection or disapproval and lose true conscience.   In the fast we feel unified with the world and always centered--a unique spirit vibrating with nature. The perception of self shifts from feeling vulnerable or tenuous to invulnerable and safe.

Your perception of self also changes: From feeling victimized and hooked to self-centered drives which degrade your self-esteem or control, to a vision of self as a perfect unique seed symbol. Just by fasting you now have superior control which is ego-less as you gain access to God.

Your perception of others is changed.   From seeing them as opportunistic, treacherous, deceitful, threatening and "different" to seeing them as simply unfolding beings--yes evil but mostly dense. The fast brings true intimacy as people now respond with interest and warmth—that's the fast-attraction. Your perception of the environment changes: from overreactions to trivia and easily being irritated with interruptions to there being no effect or strife. Here you flow with interruptions through clear instinctive reactions.

In the dense (eating) state you may feel your behavior in life must be vigilant, cautious, controlling, forceful and manipulative. In the fasting state it is relaxed and clear for your energy is upward to God not against others. It becomes an easy life of simplicity and sign-seeking: this is synchronicity as miracles fit together like a jigsaw puzzle. Your responsibility for actions and reactions is also different: from avoiding, ignoring or evading to accepting, learning and facing up to things—no more the phony surrounded by foes. You are now fearless and friendly. From having nothing but petty people-problems, fasting now gains favor with man and angels all around.

Your perception of the future changes from the sense of impending doom to always better, fuller, easier, more profound and carefree. You will even look forward to the elder state of infinite consciousness. Your inner world will go from anxiety and fear to relaxed, calm and confident well-being despite all problems. Your patterns of growth will surely change: from constant fears of victorious enemies leading to non-creativity and all energy directed against, to no competition--all energy going upward with utter fascination. In your own stream there is no competition.

Your goal-setting will change. From a tendency to limit goals and force the fit via maps and plans to setting high goals and then falling to them gently via magical interruptions created by God. What a relief to give up that compelling forceful show just to prove things to an indifferent world that could care less!   There are other black-and-white differences: Like your perceptions of power: from ambivalence to authority (admiration combined with hate) and seeing only black and white labels and status, to relating to people as they are--unimpressed with images.

The fast is the answer for the hopeless. The worse you are the more you are about to experience a metamorphosis that will shock your world. Hang on while the worst becomes the best and you overcome all obstruction in our situation. It's not a matter of how we get to cosmic consciousness but rather what keeps us from it for it is the most natural thing to have. It's not a matter of how to get up but what keeps us down. So if you're down what keeps you there? For much of the time it is food, it's effects and the habit of eating.

PEOPLE PROBLEMS

If adversity only bend a man it just makes him stronger. The biggest obstacle to genius is being ignored, misjudged and trivialized by the dense dull herd.   But the fast clears things up fast. In clarity every one and everything is novel and new. As it all comes together in beautiful wholes all we must do is watch while each moment the ever-changing puzzle fits perfectly. Then cosmic man does nothing but attract what he is, knowing that God is his only source. He has found the fast as key to this attraction: Then, since there is no time or space, past and future are here right now in the magic moment. This "collapsed" moment is pithy with solutions and witty inventions to any problem you may have. Fast to see them. Clear, your attractions stay pure and God is everywhere at all times.

What a wonderful adventure on which you are about to embark. I feel it every single morning as I face the new God-designed day. Whereas before I would eat to smudge that design now I fast and wait patiently as the miracles unfold in divine order. A crisis? Relax- -it only opens new avenues--sometimes we need to be goaded to move but it is sure to be smooth! Fasting is a shield so now our troubles must yield. In fasting we stay King and Queen. Eating for pleasure keeps us down, dense, dull and mean.

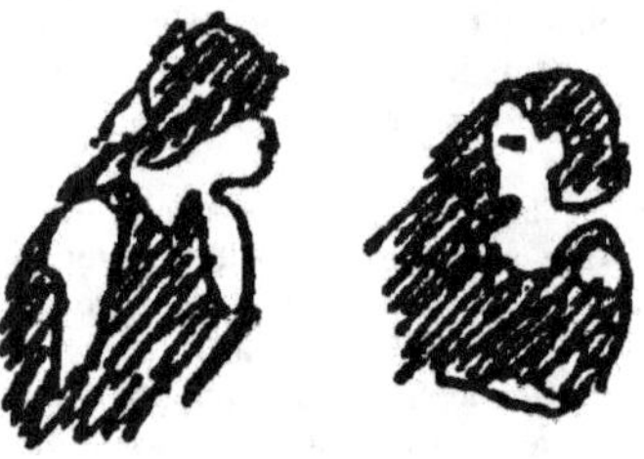

FROM PALL AND PALE
TO PANACHE AND PATINA

The two opposite states are the key to understanding what is happening in the fast and will urge you to do it more. Soon you'll look forward to and always return to it when all else fails. It will take you from pall and pale to panache and patina: Pall is to become pale, to appall, to lose strength and effectiveness, to lose interest or attraction, to become tired of something, to cause to become insipid, to satiate. Pale means to be deficient in color or intensity, not bright and brilliant but dim feeble and faint and deficient in chroma--dense energy makes one pallid. This all describes the boring and ordinary way we look and feel when eating wrong. Being pall and pale is a mighty weak impression.

Panache refers to an ornamental tuft like feathers on a helmet, dash or flamboyance in style and action, verve and nerve. You need this panache to distinguish yourself. Patina is a green film formed on copper by long exposure and valued for beauty: color. This refers to your surface appearance which grows more beautiful with age--an aura derived from habit and established character. Nothing does this better or quicker than the habit of daily fasting--mini-fasting.

FROM PALLIATION AND PAIN
TO PALATIAL AND PATHFINDING

Palliation refers to the tendency to cloak or conceal, to reduce the violence of, to abate, to cover with excuses and apologies--to constantly excuse yourself. Pain refers to payment, penalty and punishment. We certainly have paid dearly for not fasting or eating right--as the years pass the lack of success combined with fading appearance seems mentally harder to remedy. Pain refers to the unpleasant or distressing sensations due to insulin disorder: acute mental or emotional stress or suffering: grief. This describes the life of the carb-addicted procrastinator who has not completed his life's work: throes, cares, troubles, fruitless effort or exertion. And its all for naught--it could change overnight.

But then through fasting we spring to palatial: of or relating to a palace--suitable to a magnificent mansion. The word palatine is like a holy or roman emperor, the possessing of royal privileges. A feudal lord issuing sovereign power over and within his domains. Yes the fast takes us--separates us--unto the highest calling, the treasure hard (impossible) to attain through any other method. We gain access to the highest through the fast, a secret tunnel. We then become a pathfinder: one that discovers a way--a prophet, an inventor, a statesman--that's you today.

FROM PALTRINESS AND PATHOLOGY
TO PERFECTION AND   PALMS

Paltriness: inferior, trashy, mean, despicable or trivial. Do you see yourself or are you seen this way? What a horrible plight since you are actually fine--designed by God the Creator of it all. Are you pathological--caught in a disease and the structural/functional changes produced by it? Are you actually something abnormal, held down by the anatomic and physiologic deviations from the normal that make you a diseased person? I was. So much sugar and the results—compulsive food obsessions--killed my dreams. Thank God that through specific food restrictions this nightmare was dissolved. I can pass a bakery and not feel a twinge—that's all my problems resolved. I've discovered a way to live with my inborn tendencies and physical (ectomorphic) limitations regarding food so I'm no more evil-involved (along with the other addictions I used to self-medicate the constant dull drag). Having cured to the core, the whole early life trauma has been solved and each day I soar!

Fast and you'll begin a problem-free existence. If there are problems, you'll love the challenge as your spiritual sporting blood is up. Through the fast you'll attain perfection: a state of flawlessness, completeness, maturity and saintliness will take hold. You will exemplify supreme excellence and unsurpassable accuracy in your talent. Now the reward for this will be the palms: the symbol of victory and rejoicing triumph. You will be palmy: flourishing and prosperous. It will be like palm Sunday: like the palms strewn by the welcoming multitude on Christ's re-entry into Jerusalem. Yes your comeback will be that big--and it was always here as an opposing force attracted to your higher altitude through fasting.

Even if you choose the Ramadan fast where you eat first, the same things occur because now that the food is "behind" you your fasting consciousness takes over: It's your intentions that create the big shift! What a wonderful gift from God--you don't have to be the hero fasting thirty days.   Just fasting for this day is like a thousand years to the Lord who can change desire into destiny! As a daily fastarian your miracle happens today.

FASTERS ARE WINNERS, EATERS ARE WHINERS

Fasters are the winners. They can see that the eating life is constant cravings, a futile fix that has no fruition--it just repeats itself without solving problems or bringing you joy (the delusion for which you are doing it). Eating is only lust--the taste trip. While the herd eats, they talk of the next meal, the next restaurant and this lust veils the backlash of suffering later. Now that is true addiction--craving the fix without thoughts of the horror that comes afterward. It's a lifestyle that costs dearly. It took me years to realize how much happier I was without even the right food. I loved the higher mental life--which instantly dissolves through food's fix. We can't have both. My first mini-fast was the happiest day of my life. After one fatty meal I had a most miraculous right-brained day with God. In this state I learned to see all delays as the fastest route and all "crises" as the answer to prayer. Sometimes at night I may have some fruit and sleep so cozily waking up in the arms of God, fully cleansed and ready for the new day.

RIDING AIR CURRENTS

Fasting on sun and air will change your chemistry, tissues and every cell.   The metamorphosis is a striking alteration in appearance, character or circumstances defined as a "marked or abrupt change in form and structure subsequent to birth or hatching." Fasting precedes conversion. It is also a metaplasia: a transformation of one tissue into another, or metasomatism--the changing of the chemical composition as well as the texture of "rock." One's entire body, tissues, bloodstream and cells are changed suddenly. To substantiate this change in my outer circumstances I kept a "fasting miracles" diary. It listed an otherworldly, uncanny, impossible set of miracles which occur on a fast. These are things so coincidental that they could never happen again. The daily miracles for a month were incomprehensible--there was nothing subtle about them. I saw giant debt-cancellations, purchases arriving two weeks early, seeing childhood friends after dreaming of them and many other "magic coincidences".

After a while I happened to go back to eating regularly and the miracles stopped as I lost the fasting spirit or fasting consciousness. I went back into the same old boredom, compulsive craving and bleak perception. The miraculous co-ordination left and I became out-of-sync making stupid mistakes and feeling disordered. Then three months later I suddenly had a glimpse of the difference, made the switch and came back into fasting and the daily miracles (the "spirit of fasting"). The switch is automatic in the marvelous body-instrument. Walking out in the beautiful desert in the brightest light on earth--there is no greater joy. As I walk all day with five dogs no one can involve me in worldly entertainment for it pales in comparison to the Godly elements--the elemental reality. Gross nutrition (starches, sugars, food concoctions and inventions) is just a hook as it lures and then traps us down. It never works but only swells the abdomen, holds useless water and makes our wake-up turgid and slow. Only the elements bring spiritual bliss.

THE   WORST   DAY   PRECEDES   THE   BEST

The day before you look your best you look your worst as the earliest layers of tough crud from ancient storage kicks out to the glorious rebirth of trillions of cells. Just before this occurs the mirror shows ugly revenge of years of wrong eating. From a young age I wanted to improve myself. As an artist I noticed that candle light and shadows reflected bad proportions on a sick face in contrast to the carved and sharp features of a healthy body and blood. If eating right we see the magic face of the True Self. People peg your present personality by the configuration of your face! With pasty-sugary carb old pals say "she's never changed, she's still crazy." And they are right--because when not eating right we bloat down to lower levels where we fall into stereotypic perception--culturally-defined meanings of things. The dulled mind falls in with the majority as here genius meets a hard wall as the wind is kicked out of its sails. Only fasting and the right diet elevates us above hostile backgrounds and people by separating us from society, sick systems and cycles of sin.

Fasting resolves the clash between left and right, nature and society, God and culture. Fasting is the mainstay of the new life, the device to stay close to God as the talents come through with "holy spirit ease." Forget compulsive meditation for if eating wrong nothing endures. Fasting always works as fear dispels and truth alights. "Where there is no vision people perish." Vision is lost when the engine dysfunctions and degenerates in the compacted state of carb-storage--and vision arrives when this obstruction dissolves. The carb-hodgepodge creates a toxic personality veiled by image. It isn't the meat-eaters who are in a rage--it's the carb-addicts feeling caged!

GOD   BLESSES   THE   FAST
Skin and Lymph

Keep thinking: "God blesses the fast. Only He knows all." You have no idea how fast the fast will change you. The sky's the limit as your new face opens doors: From a broad-faced square-jawed "fortiesh-fiftiesh" look to a thin ageless jawline. When square-faced people instantly peg you with cruel ageist comments. Thin-faced and ageless the same people adoringly hang on to your every word, as the new archetype cues the counter-script. The true issue is: eating wrong brings prejudice. For women aging is hard but the new regime will erase all these mid-life problems of persecution, pain and procrastination. The irritability, stupor, brain fog, insomnia and anger from carbs will forever hold you back-- you are "dead" as all doors close along with your arteries. Fat evokes glucagons which dilates the arteries while sugar and starch evokes insulin which closes them down. Fat-fast and all systems dilate and the future says "Go!"

Skin Brushing. The skin is a seven-pound eliminative organ. When fasting so much comes out each pore. Expect chapping, bumps and rashes as this dissolving and realignment occurs-- for your skin will look aged first, then suddenly "youthified" as the lymph and blood again runs clear. My whole body was filled with itchy bumps for twenty-four hours, then the next morning all smoothed out and all wrinkles were gone. Expect pus, boils and pustules formed of micro-organisms, mucus and tissue debris.   Brush the skin twice daily. It will feel like your "scratching" every pore as sudden lymph cleansing is evoked and   the next day's stool shows sticky lymph fluid and pus. It's an amazing but simple trick that you will love as you see sand floating through the air: evoking the dumping of storage pockets of debris and fat.

MINI-FASTING

The mini-fast is eating once only and then flying off to a 23 hour fast every single day. This regime becomes easier as each day one is cleaner, clearer and more joyous. Digestion, assimilation and elimination become more efficient each and every day. The found time between each meal is so creative (the consciousness of God being pure rapture and delight) that the 23 hours will fly by quickly with no thoughts of food. Some people find it easier to eat the meal mid-day with skipping breakfast and dinner a snap. Eat a nice big meal so you won't feel deprived. I always prefer digestion in the early mornings to maximize the impact of air and sun during the day and to be ready for everything and anything in the business-public forum without ever being seen eating. Begin with raisins (grapecure) or figs (unless fat-fasting) and end with avocado or fauna fat--that satisfies and makes fasting a snap and happy song. Look forward, it won't be long!

NO MORE BAD HAIR DAYS

Women often speak of the depression going with "bad hair days". Well fasting determines everything from the part in your hair, the proportions of the face, the skeletal alignment. Now talk to the cameras! No more bloated planes, just a fine crystal--perfectly even, taut, tight, happy and childlike. If eating right the years have no bearing on the face. If eating wrong rapid aging is a given. A healthy face will open doors for you, a bloated face will shut them just as fast. Stay even now. For the older you are the more your downs will show drastically. People will love you one day and be fearfully disappointed in you the next. Age demands you stay even! The true champion is ever-up and never-down.

Do it once.   You'll be so happy you'll do it everyday. Its like exercise—you must break into it to enjoy it as a habit. At first the notion of daily fasting seems so empty and boring. But then when you "eat the universe" how vastly different and varied your experience becomes. You must achieve this experience as the fast brings you favor with the world. The average binger who avoids fasting will be the one to experience the greatest transformation when finally doing it. Go towards your greatest fears--to release your greatest power.

To mini-fast, eat one big meal. This is best for the colon works on the principal of mass evacuation. One big meal--what excuse would anyone have for eating again? Many "fruitarians" eat all day. Anyone can eat fruit but no one wants to fast. This mini-fast regimen combines both in every day. As the Bible says "fast and pray daily." Eating once is spectacular. Eating twice is not bad if the two meals are six hours apart leaving 18 hours of fasting each day. For the neophyte that too will be spectacular as the results are cumulative.

Fasting teaches you to appreciate the eternally beautiful things--seeing poetry everywhere. Whenever something is not quite right just fast into eternity. Step into your future--create new realities, love yourself, watch and observe all. You will always be better off fasting, enjoying reality at a higher level. You'll soon learn how to appreciate the fasting process as guilt, fear and shame dissolve. Fasting erases or beautifies the past, present and future. No matter what one did you're now fasting and that settles it--you're free (or soon will be). A faster never says he's fasting--why tell them his bag of tricks? He could easily lose the fasting spirit so he never gambles with it.

NEW YEARS EVERY DAY

The big thing about New Years is the opportunity to start a brand new life and forget the old as if it never were. Similarly each time one fasts it's like a re-baptism. A faster--the King or Queen--becomes a universal archetype, not a cultural family or gender stereotype. You're free--and always the sun--Egyptian sultan, shaman, Indian priest, happy dusky child. You'll look like eternity, a carved face on a coin or the moon. The wise ones will know you from experience—you're the eternity they all know, represented in one ever-changing symbol.

For the power of correct vision just say "I'll be famous today" or "God will reward me for not eating when everyone else is eating." With each hunger pain more beauty will result as cells uncramp and spill their contents into the bloodstream going through. Soon you'll see a prettier face. Today is the day you unhook from the human herd you know--the beasts attempting to argue you down--and you reject their stuff along with the food. You're with angels, animals, ancestors and the Great Mind of all the greatest discoverers that ever lived. Do an experiment: begin fasting then sit down to a desk facing nature. Grab a pen and paper and wait. Soon an outpouring of primal truths about your own and God's nature will be released--to your great relief.   These new truths will settle all doubts while they reveal your good points and the blocks to success. Now just fast and wait for the mass attractions coming soon. With every hunger pain denied God rewards the ride. Soon you'll hit the highest tide, a whirlwind success bonafide.

THE FAST IS THE END

Now THE END occurs--the completion of old cycles and the beginning of new ones. Fast and you'll become more energetically childlike every day. The minute your work is complete there's a gravitational pull to materialize it on earth. It took you decades to form the kernel which now attracts pollination. Rest assured that your completion forms this kernel-cue creating the True End--the blessings of the new life of due recognition. As your self-expression hits the mark it makes an amazing new dent in the world--the Revitalization of Culture.

16

LACTO-FRUITARIANS

Free of Deficiency: Fruit and Cheese

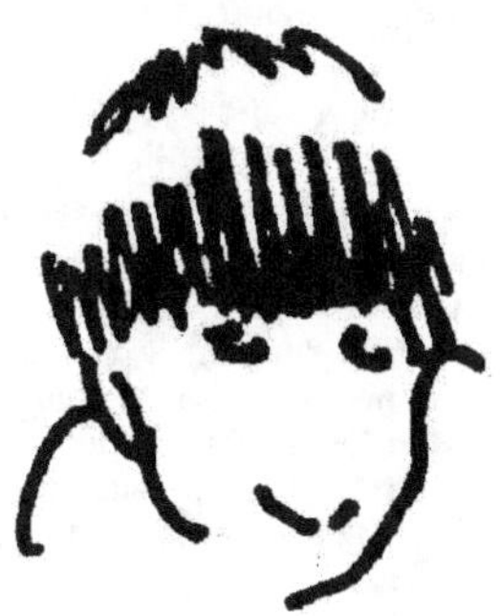

Ever heard of a "peaches 'n cream" complexion? This is lacto-fruitarianism.   The subject of this chapter is the effects of not enough protein. Lacto-fruitarianism is a good compromise ensuring freedom from deficiency while allowing you to stay on a predominantly fruit and fasting diet. A fig and later a piece of cheese—what could be easier? Humans are omnivorous--they are fat-frugivores: animal food-eaters who also eat fruit. Man needs animal protein and longterm fruitarian/vegans usually suffer from deficiencies. But there are those among you who just cannot eat meat--you can't get beyond the "animal-on-the-plate" and neither can I.   But if one lived on a small farm with a goat, taking care of her in exchange for sustenance would be a normal way to live. If you wish to remain fruitarian a little cheese is the way to do it.   For me a long-term fruitarian who had the habit of eating crates of grapes and dates, the tendency towards hyper-insulinism was so great that for awhile just one piece of fruit brought on headaches, nervousness, moodiness, cravings and constricted breathing. After one year of fat-fasting with one cheese omelet a day this all stabilized so now I can assume my fat-frugivorous status--the original and best diet of man. My basic diet became raisins, figs, pineapple, cheese and cashews with 18 hours fasting daily. Having overcome the dead duo of protein deficiency and insulin resistance the body revived, the mind restored and my work came out. The FTT problem--the failure to thrive—was gone!

LACTO-FRUITARIANS

Lacto-fruitarianism refers to fruitarianism with dairy products for protein and fat. Now dairy is not paleo--it's regarded as agricultural. But milk and cheese precede the farming age by at least 20,000 years (Billings) and as animal foods they are still fat and far exceed beans and grains in health benefits as the former are dangerous to the immune system—they "make no sense" to the body which only responds to the logic of fauna and fruit. Cheese is much older than agriculture as the nomadic goat-herders throughout the world used it as a way of storing milk for the winter.   The ancient Greek Olympiads were put on exclusive cheese diets.   When I eat cheese it's store-bought because the raw organic creates body-pain in anyone who is mold-sensitive. (Another raw vegan myth exploded.)

DIET DOGMA IS DESTRUCTIVE

The lesson: Dogma kills. "Reason" kills. The bigger lesson: we cannot listen to anyone--they're all hypnotized by whatever the current dogma is. I cannot stress this point enough. They may be enmeshed in a previous matrix made obsolete by a new one. Never forget the characteristic of any scientific pre-revolutionary era is confusion, masked by phobic superstitions and myth! What one person sees as "mucus-production" (bad), another sees as "adequate protein" (good). Man loves nuts, but invariably there is someone who says "don't eat too many—they're so fatty".   Yet for some people the more nuts they eat the better the elimination because the colon needs fat and fiber.   Whatever you think, the opposite could be the truth or some fact you never thought of. But what I had to go through for years because I listened to anything other than my own instincts. I love fat. I regard my fat-stash as my rejuvenator for the month, my staff, my mainstay. As an anorexic (ectomorph) I was never given avenues to deal with the problem of full-phobia and having to stay thin to be able to breath properly. I had to invent this diet, to be cured for good of all anorexic tendencies and still fast which every instinct says to do. I was never told how to eat to stay stable--I had to discover a way, and this is yours today. Stick to the cheese tray and throw all your beans and rice away—and don't give it to your dogs or their health will also pay.

RASTAFARIAN FRUITARIANS

Rastafarian fruitarians are those who eat fish for protein and fat (fish oils). Jesus fasted forty days but he also ate fish. This is an important food model as many fruitarians never fast (they can be gluttons of fruit or avocados) and many refuse to eat protein foods of any kind just to maintain the false fruitarian ideology that "all one needs is 1.5% protein just like mother's milk." It works so well at first--it brings a haunting beauty as the eyes roll back in the head in a "yin" way and it makes one feel "spiritual" and close to God as he feels he has the keys to the universe. But slowly and so insidiously things turn. As the body fails the ego buttresses up the diet as "superior " to compensate. People turn away as the ego grows and there is more isolation. Then trouble starts as he refuses to see doctors. This chapter is on the harmful effects of this protein deficiency to work against this circuitous mental reaction. However you get it, eat protein and fat. Add fish, cheese or eggs to the diet then fast 18 hours and all health will restore. You'll say of this lifestyle: " I want more, and will never close this door."

PROTEIN DEFICIENCY

Fruitarians suffer with extreme deficiency symptoms from protein malnourishment--the biggest effect being a suppressed immune system. In the 60's and 70's vegetarianism became popular and people deleted meat and dairy in their diet--to be replaced by foods with much less protein, much more carb in substitute and some inferior (plant-based and evolutionarily discordant) substitutions like beans and rice. At that time environmental illness (EI) also became evident and has since become pandemic--a severely compromised immune system from mass protein malnourishment.   Having low immunity they also evidence many food intolerances when attempting to include more protein and fat in their diet as evinced in bloated legs and stomach and other signs of protein malnourishment. They need to start slowly to eat fat and protein in whatever source they can tolerate--to boost immunity or die. One has reached a point--or soon will--where carbs won't work to bring normalcy and thus they show symptoms of failure to thrive.   Let's look at other symptoms of protein malnourishment:

NO MORE PINK CLOUD

"The honeymoon is over" says beyondveg.com. Look at some of the deficiency symptoms: severe muscle cramps, especially leg cramps from calcium deficiency. Then there is the dental: severe tooth erosion from acid fruit (enamel hypoplasia), and acid reflux--ever wonder why you have it when you're supposedly eating right? Then there are the sugar problems: fatigue highs/blues, excess urination and constant thirst. The fruitarian develops acute hyper-sensitivity--he can smell everything and everyone and so continues to isolate. The worst is the constant hunger and cravings, the social isolation and the fatigue. He has a big meal with plenty of avocados and he's hungry and tired a couple hours later leading to eating throughout the day. I can eat a few nuts and a slice of cheese and forget about food for the day while the fruitarian keeps eating and it irritates his non-fruit peers. To him I would ask: is it not more "pure" to eat a few nuts or some cheese to last ten hours, not needing anything else and directing your energies to some other activity?

RASTAFARIAN, LACTO- OR OVO- FRUITARIANS

Man needs fat and protein. The anti-protein argument of fruitarians that we need no more protein than mother's milk is false. The fruitarian does well for awhile just adding fruit-fat or nuts, but soon they find total rejuvenation by going Rastafarian (adding fish), lacto (dairy), or ovo (eggs).   Protein malnourishment so suppresses the immune system that soon no protein food can be eaten without severe edema. One should not take it this far--for before he's aware of it he's mistaking brain fog for hyper-spirituality. I became fruitarian to overcome the sick systems around me at the very time I needed protein to deal with the oppression. But hypnotized by dogma, I doggedly kept on in my pursuit of fruitarian purity and became frailty-- while losing all sanity.

SYMPTOMS OF FAILURE TO THRIVE

Billings lists of several symptoms of failure to thrive on raw or vegan diets: insomnia or disturbed sleep, a run-down feeling, chronically tired, very little energy, sleepy during the day, lack of normal motivation for regular daily tasks, no joy of living, hunger all the time, obsessed with eating and all-day eating, lost sex drive, frequent respiratory problems from lowered immunity and reactive nervous systems subject to upset--all the while touting fruit philosophy.

It is the "frog in boiling water" syndrome: the initial improvement is followed by long-term decline without knowing it in the "initially-better-but-followed-by-slow-decline-syndrome". One thinks "how can things end up so bad when they started out so good?" At first one goes into detox and feels so much better: everyone improves so they can't believe it can ever go sour.   Then after reserves are exhausted they decline into deficiencies which are not your typical "deficiency-disease" symptoms--but are subtly and slowly debilitating.

The fruitarian "lulling effect of imperceptibly" masks health decline.   But from a psychological standpoint this syndrome's most interesting aspect is the mental adjustment to the lowered state of health without being able to perceive it as such since they do not want to believe it is happening. They see these symptoms as the "need for more detox". Though their friends and family see otherwise they're in denial until the problems reach an undeniable point, like hospitalization.   It is emotional certainty that shuts down rational assessment of symptoms. Because of initial improvement they are so thoroughly convinced of the entire detox theory that they are now psychologically invested in the rightness of it. The detox theory is so self-consistent logically that "the willingness to make sober judgments of current symptoms is perpetually displaced into the future." The present problems are just a "temporary setback"--its either detox or detox that needs to occur. Or "the better you get the more energy to expel toxins and the more powerful the healing crises." They are more concerned about "eating right" than the actual results. The logic captivates and satisfies more than actual results.

Those who really do get good results are more "certain" than the others and thus become the "repositories of traditional wisdom" for the "superior diet" of which they can blame others for not following the details, thus reinforcing the tendency not to see failures as proof the diet is wrong. None can tolerate threats to their beliefs and this "shared ideal binds the successes and failures together in common cause. The less successful imbibe the certainty of the more successful to maintain the faith." The favored paradigm shuts down openness to new interpretations or explanations. In order to prove the system works, people redouble their efforts at detox through an even stricter diet or solve their deficiencies through even smaller details within the matrix of the same diet.

VEGAN DOGMA VS. THE REAL FACTS

Humans are omnivores, specifically fat-frugivores as indicated by the fossil record and the comparative gut anatomy and physiology of metabolism. Humans like dogs and cats are not natural vegetarians at all. Man is not a folivore—a leaf or plant-eater, for that requires a big gut for bacterial putrefaction. Plant foods are poor sources of EFAs and other long-chain fatty acids suggesting adaptation to foods including preformed long-chain fatty acids found in animal flesh. Also the slow conversion of beta-carotene to Vitamin A suggests they ate preformed vitamin A in meat. Evolutionary plant foods were poor zinc and iron sources, two essential minerals only in animal foods. Grains provide them but as products of agriculture contain anti-nutrients that inhibit mineral absorption.

The actual diets of all the great apes include meat or insects, and paleo (pre-Edenic) man ate mostly animal foods. Humans are classic examples of omnivores in all relevant anatomical traits. The best arguments for a meat-free diet remain ecological, ethical and philosophical. The vegan community condemn all omnivore diets as bad or like the SAD (standard American diet) which is so poorly filled with modern processed foods. One cannot compare the natural paleo-omnivore diet with the modern diet filled with machine processed foods.

LOVE ANIMALS!

We should love animals and one reason is because we need them for sustenance. Does this imply cruelty? No—just the opposite. It should mean we should revolutionize the dairy and meat industry to insure human methods. This new information should be a humane movement, not a degeneration into barbarism like many vegans fear it will. Actually, veganism has lowered the life vibration of the animal kingdom. For example, vegans give their dogs low fat diets, which are cruel. Give your dogs cheese and other fauna products, along with good quality dry chunks. The dogs of vegans living on vegetables and grains— and end up fat, dry, without sheen or personality. Watch them come alive on the Cheese diet--when dead logs become shiny, bouncy and youthful dogs. Further, because vegans want to eliminate dairy because of inhumane methods, the problem remains unsolved. By seeing it as man's only salvation, we can focus on humane methods—and love the animal kingdom with gratitude! Give the goat or cow pasture and protection from predators, in return for your very life sustenance. That's the old-fashioned way, the only way for today. In the meantime, just enjoy your store-bought cheese, as much as you please—and regain your youth as you finally have the keys.

BE READY

Be ready for gainsayers as they rebel against your two main concepts of (1) fat and (2) fat-fasting. They'll be against fat because they're the herd who can't think deeply. They'll be against fasting because they're the herd who can't give up their carnal comforts. It's a Dionysian generation so remember your humility is the protection from deception! The fruit and veggie crowd is filled with pride, and pride will not receive instruction and is susceptible to deception--"eat all fruit to be gods" Not only pride but the continuous insulin-elevation brings anger, envy and greed which goes with gluttony--eating fruit all day and never being satisfied. Remember the characteristics of deception: something that seems so true--but isn't.

Be ready for hostility when you speak the truth, for the "harmless" get angry because (1) they've given up animal foods when their inner instincts really desire it and (2) constantly elevated insulin creates emotional instability and moodiness.   Insulin aggravates hypertension by increasing the responsiveness of the arteries to the effects of adrenaline (jungle mentality of shooting at shadows) just as it effects the neurotransmitters causing sleep disorders and next-day moods.

THIS END IS YOUR BEGINNING

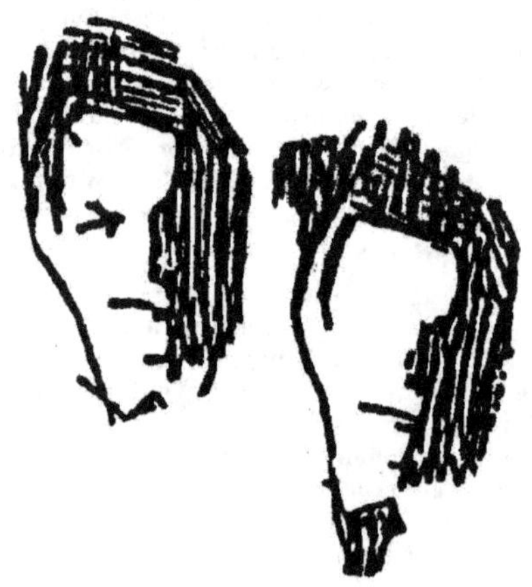

I'm asking you to take this new science knowledge and modify it for your needs--this is wisdom. The main points are the necessity of the high-protein fat diet and the fact that it's not fat that makes you fat but carb. The fat-fast works so efficiently to eliminate fat from your body and food from your thought-life--to then "fill" it with a new life of witty inventions and creative action! Get this, become a whole new person and then ignore all your critics. As the highest on the phylogenetic ladder you were designed to eat fat, fruit and to fast.

FAT FASTING REGIME
And Elimination

This is a major switch but your body is going to adapt beautifully. When the one-week adaptation is over you will quite happily be living on one small fat-protein or fat meal a day. Those without hyperinsulinism may go right to the FFF diet with figs, raisins (grapecure), nuts and cheese or other types of fauna. I suggest you fast in the evening (just skip dinner) for if fasting, human growth hormone elevates at night which perfects the engine (youthifies). Your monthly food bill will be low, you will never be hungry and you will be super-healthy with low cholesterol. Your breathing will be better than ever.   A note on elimination: whether you take a salad or psyllium husks as a bulking agent is up to you. I prefer the natural bulk of these foods to herbal preparations—especially the black fruit and nuts but also the cheese since the colon needs fat. But for the beginner (bogged down by feces) let me say that as a 21st century high-tech diet, psyllium husks will complete the fruit-fat-fastarian diet.

For the first three days on the fat-fast you may feel very good. Your body is getting the fat and protein it needs unencumbered with carb which completely confuses things. Then you'll be no-hunger fasting which also feels so good. But then on the fourth through the sixth day your body sees it may be living this way for some time and goes through adaptation. Your enzymes are experiencing a "changing of the guard." You may experience fatigue, mild depression, brain fog and a loss of fascination experienced on the first three days. This is also due to glucagon's burning up of debris from years going through the bloodstream. On the seventh day--the end of the first week--things begin to change. You see a much younger person in the mirror with taut smooth skin and a much narrower face and head indicating youth. You feel very even--you may not feel like yourself when you were "hyper" which you labeled "energetic." This is a mild, smooth, even calm and poised regal temperament of "aristocratic reserve." Wait out this first week, expect a couple foggy days and then prepare for the end result: feeling good all the time, devoid of highs and lows just mild calm and even energy. You'll be amazed at your lack of hunger and you won't think of eating again after the one meal. Congratulations! You have now fasted for one week and you're on your way to a brand new rich life met through moist skin and clear mind. Judge for your self when ready to add more fruit: You'll know the time is right/wrong by the presence/absence of insulin's symptoms.

17

FRUITS OF FASTING STARS

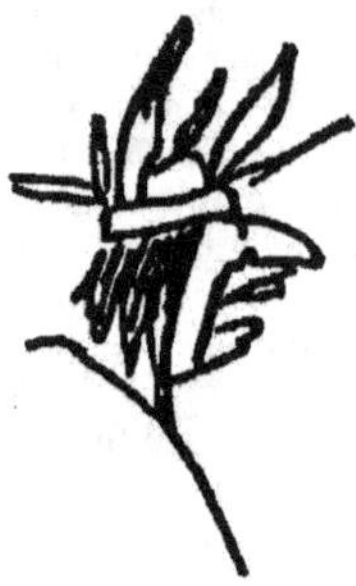
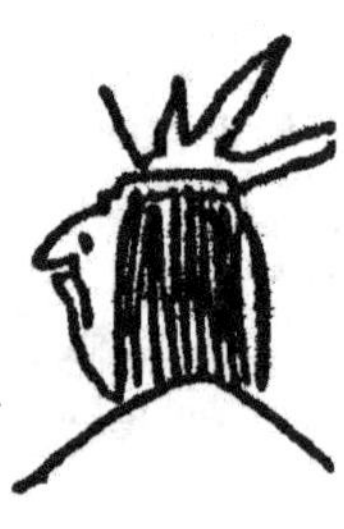

GABBING AND GORGING

Gabbing and gorging go together. Gabbers talk to much, habitually and idly. This describes the human race who lives to eat, sleep and "socialize." The three go together. Not the faster--he loves silence so he can communicate with God, the One who matters. He prefers fasting to stay high in the head with continuous revelation and he needs only recharging catnaps, not so much sleep. The eater eats to bring energy down out of the head to avoid facing himself. It's a temporary way of dealing with low self-esteem: to deaden the brain by lowering it to the stomach. Eating is the "best" distraction which works instantly. To eradicate this tendency we'll look at the stuff of everyday man vs. the Fruits of the Fasting Stars.

Everyday man doesn't just talk--he gabbles: this is talking fast and foolishly, jabbering like a "gabby"--a simpleton. He likes to gab-gatte---be on the go to little purpose but to serve his fruitless desires. He's a gadabout---a person who flits about in social activity with other gaderenes--demon-possessed swine that rush into the sea. They're all gadflies---flies that bite and annoy, stirring up other people just to soothe their restless spirits. When everyday man is finally alone he quickly focuses on TV, for just music isn't enough. He must intensely focus his whole being, eyes and ears on another reality other than his own.

What does a person do if left alone on an island? At first he may panic but then with time begins to unravel the outer layers and come to himself (alone in nature, man clears). In retreating inward he comes to feel part of nature--the true inner meets the outer as the phony fades away. At that juncture he begins to feel intense happiness for the first time in his life.

When eating the wrong food one becomes an entirely different person--in looks, speech, thoughts and character. The lower state attracts gaff: a hoax, fraud, gimmicks, tricks, rough treatment, abuse and social blunders. To avoid faux pas he is gagged: his mouth is stopped up with something inserted (the foot or food).   But the bad food creates autonomisms (out-of-control slips of the tongue). Gag is also the censure of other people with whom one eats, for the "social eating society" prevents free speech. This is the gag rule restricting freedom of expression as one must not talk too deep--dinner conversation must be light and non-threatening!   Eating soothes the feelings of rejection from this censure. You can't talk but you can eat--it's a trade-off.

Gaga means crazy, foolish and infatuated--another side of the eating fool. Like all addicts he falls in love suddenly but it doesn't last long. The couple eats together as they fall in love--eating becomes the system--but it dies as love is dulled with blood-irritants (but if she's a good cook it lasts longer). Gageg is a token of defiance and a pledge of combat as pugnacity prevails from insulin-elevating foods and other irritants leading to insane moodiness. Gaiety refers to their merrymaking gay spirits as the epicureans chat and eat (for tomorrow they die).

Then there are the fat-fasters living on highest quality (HQ) food along with air and sun. They show gain: to win in competition and conflict by natural development or process. They achieve: traverse, cover, attract attention, profit and increase while improving in health. This is becoming a "heavy"--to run fast and get gain! These are the fat-fasters eating the correct food for man and then living with God while high in the head. They are gainful : "I will increase as you decrease." Yes austerity has great rewards. Gainly is the graceful, shapely and perfect shape constellated from fat-and-fruit-fed iron red blood.

Now if one slips back to culture-food he encounters gainsay: to be spoken against and contradicted. This is the constant plight from wrong eating--all one says or does meets great resistance. When he returns to the right way he is   gaited--having a fancy gait and a new spring in his step. He is now galactic---of the galaxy, a Galahad--like a knight finding the fountain of youth. One resembles a galatea: an ivory statue of a beautiful maiden. One's beauty will now be created by God after being on this potter's wheel of fasting and the correct food. Let it happen--no pain no gain. You're now created by nature, a galax--an evergreen herb with decorative leaves. Clean, you'll now catapult up to the galax: an assemblage of brilliant and notable persons through time.   No more gale-emotional outbursts from protein/fat deprivation and the incorrect food. You're under complete self-control due to and reflected in your austere eating habits.   And no more galimatias: confused and meaningless talk like gibberish or gall: bitterness of spirit, irritation or harassment.

The mistake of thinking that energy comes from food is so engrained that fatigue often leads fruitlessly to fake food which leads to more fatigue and craving. We get hungry because we eat things that elevate insulin--one little bit and the craving starts. The idea of fasting is so simple: reduce the burden on the body and it snaps back into perfect shape. Fast and energy is saved to perfect the body instead, working much like a computer: when you turn it off it returns to "factory settings." Maturity is learning four important things: what to eat, when to eat, when not to eat and when to fast.

BE A RARE SPARKLING PERSON

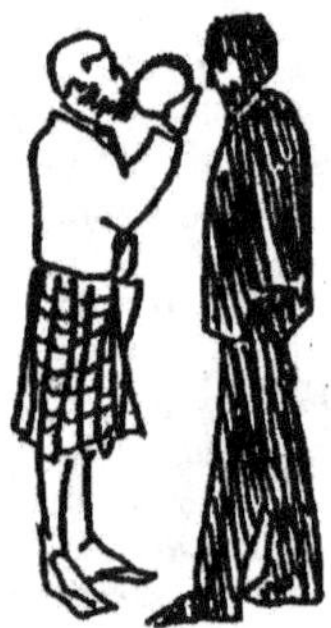

Much of the reason to fast is social. At the basis of wrath is bowel-toxicity projected onto others who have bowel toxicity. When clear of carb-laden foods and fat we become a rare sparkling person. You must have the shine to be fine—to have luster divine. That sparkle of divinity comes from fat—the spirit-conducting oil—and the fast.   The would-be saint is always victimized for being "different", on the fringe, the outcast. But fast and all that changes. You'll feel so good with each break-fast meal as the fat just continues the glucagons-elevated fast.

TIMES OF DAY: ROUTINE

What a joy to live intensely in the times of day and the seasons in line with nature. First you rise in joy. Then eat, enjoy and digest as God's fat and oil exhilarates the tissues. Now the fun begins. Yoga—stretch, elongate, realign to supreme relief and the big "shift" (from worldly resentments and pastimes to the spirit of God--the "anointing"). Sun--it feels so good on fat-nourished skin as it is absorbed so deep into the cells of the fasting body. Then fresh air metabolizes as it energizes. Fasting and prayer creates a blissful afternoon in communication with God, breathing fresh air from the country. Now you have deep sleep: as glucagons opens everything up it is better than ever—blissful, deep, happy, comfy with no cravings. A traumatized person from the wrong metabolism becomes "ugly", but eat the fat of the land and fast—then all the lines sooth to moist smoothness again. Just live each day in this Godly manner and you'll be most interested in the spiritual world, free of all stress no matter what is happening in the physical. Unplug from the lusty crowd who can't get enough food and attain the spiritual skies instead!

EVEN FRUITARIANS MUST FAST

By not eating you're doing so much. Deprived of the energy burden of digestion, the body snaps back into perfect shape. You've now won the right of nature's protection--no harm comes to the fat-fastarian who also eats fruit. This is the perfection of well-oiled "regina beauty". It's a serious decision which one can't lie about--there are no fat-fasters with wrinkles! The lacto-fruitarian fat-faster is protected by mother nature herself through the cow or goat. This natural relationship is your new mother—magna mater—and it's a perfect old-fashioned dyad. Take good care of that (symbolic) animal and she will take care of you in the most soothing and calming way through the provision of fat.

RESEMBLE A SHINY POT

You must resemble a shiny pot. Once there, don't slip back into starchy concoctions or you'll fail worse than ever. Once having been "oiled", putting carb-sand on the new baby tissue brings the greatest fat-storage ever. Once you fast and get into the higher eliminative forces of air, sun, prayer, yoga and are fueled by the wonderful aspects of fat and protein described throughout this book as well as getting much needed rest (which often means isolation) you won't believe you waited so long to give up all that food and the "eating life". Fast and tell no one--for people will bring you down. How did the devil tempt Jesus? By luring him into eating bread. Without fasting there is only degeneration and dishonor. Fast to let there be light. Fast for the fruits of a True Star!

ECTOMORPHY: BODY MYSTICISM

The muscular (mesomorph) man puts his faith in the muscular system (striking power and defense). The fat man (endomorph) puts his faith in food and the digestive system as the only means of survival. The thin man (ectomorph) puts his faith in the sensory system. He knows that food only degrades his perceptions, the "high" spirituality he feels when free of food. All my life I felt very strange in this land of big people who thought so very differently from myself. There are two separate nervous systems and two brains. When free of digestion the brain automatically shifts to the right, to the cornucopia where miracles fit together in the here-and-now. Here the past collapses as the future arrives. I love this state--it's exactly why fasting precedes the conversion process.

The Italian school of Clinical Anthropology calls the ectomorph an hyper-evolute--hyper meaning above and over, further along in evolution. It is much more evolved to live off what you sense and perceive rather than gross food or fighting. The skinny ectomorph is so evolved he looks futuristic as his elevation in consciousness is furthered by his body. I call this concept (of the integration of mind and body) "body mysticism". He has found God in his body by luminizing his tissues. This gives him total self-control without thinking about it--he prefers the higher spiritual life and has learned that eating drugs it out of sight. Any new obstruction triggers the left-brain--a pale, gray roadmap of reality. He simply wants to be up, not down wearing a frown.

Properly nourished on fat then fasting is a proprioceptive sensory journey from which the ectomorph never wants to return.   Despite collision with culture (or the big, dominant and mean) the rewards are a regular routine in the reality of the thin with sheen! I was a sickly sallow anorexic and then a scrawny sad fruitarian. Now I'm a sturdy sanguine fat-faster, happily skinny. No more sapped, this way is safe!

FUTURISTIC FRUIT-FAT-FASTARIANISM

Fat-fasting combines the glories of fasting with high-tech science about what to eat. The fruit and fat needs are the most important. The fatarian or fat-frugivore lives his life creatively as a spiritual scientist, conforming to no one--he is related to the universal energy source and connects upward in continuous revelation from God. This is facilitated by a ketone-loving brain and bloodstream. He relates vertically to God through the conductivity of divine talents but not so much horizontally to man: he just brings things through for materialization on earth. He does not act against in competition nor does he act with in conformity but remains fixed in the Inner Journey. If he ever does return to dense stimulation and lower pleasures he suffers greatly (more than the others) and returns to the right path quickly. Being thin his energy is higher and he clears faster.

RESEMBLE A CHISOLED CHILD SO MILD

As he matures he learns about his body differences and never looks back. Due to the higher paleo diet his face takes on the carved chiseled strength of a wise old man who looks ten (like Ghandi). His skin is lustrous and he is agelessly free of superfluity in his delicate, wiry, hyper-sensitive and high-powered engine so perfectly adapted to his new champion life of spiritual light, wisdom and power. The other two types (the muscular mesomorph and fat endomorph) are anachronistic mal-adaptations to the early era of materialism: controlling and socializing. The era of materialism is also of addiction: gabbing, gorging, accumulating, storing, hording, fighting, debating, conquering, invading, self-aggrandizing, recovering and dying slowly from the sad effects.

Become now a gentle ectomorphic saint and everything will reverse for you like dominoes. Fasting and a happy congenial body overcomes all network prejudices and herd obstacles as they'll all say "she was a saint all along." To be a success just plant all the seeds, be silent and fast as all obstacles are overcome. Those who profess nobility must fight for that image--so can you fast? If you can the unseen presence and the angels are now revealed and firm in mind. Don't worry over decades of unremunerated work--you will now end that preparatory journey by fasting in pure "rich" delight: Via the fat-fast the sun, moon, stars and due recognition (and remuneration) will soon be yours.

SIGNS OF THE NEED FOR FASTING

Whenever you feel these things fast or age into uselessness: lack of energy, tiredness, irritability, restlessness, intolerance, quarrelsomeness, fatigue, lack of endurance, body odor, constipation, despair, bad skin, self-doubt, any illness or failure. Are you nostalgically brooding over things that are gone and can never return? Are you steeped in the past—does it occupy your mind like an obsession? That's a lost life and you need to transcend the physical world through fasting. Your fears of aging or loosing people will dissolve. You need a higher world to live where all these problems and past-times go "strangely dim." A higher world exists and awaits your membership—enter it today to escape the usual human horrors. Fill your cave with storable items—nuts, figs, hard green apples or cans of pineapple, olives, raisins—and then fast without fears of lack or spoilage. I don't want a bunch of fresh fruit around that I must "eat lest it spoil". I go for dried and canned—in this home fresh fruit's been banned and despite what "rawists" say on the pinnacle of health I stand! Both the fast and the feast-potential (the sense of abundance that won't wither or waste) will start you on your new fat-fastarian life of miraculous surprises and happy coincidences planned by God for His saints.

HOMELY, LONELY AND BORED?
Try a Fig Fast

The more deformed, homely and ugly the more elastic you are and the more beautiful you'll be soon. Take this on faith first, then make a before-and-after photo to prove it. Fasting will be your friend from that point on, so move on. You're removing a ton, and it means mon. Get out in the son, and walk briskly—move those parts for champion power off the charts. Follow these books on the paleo-fasting arts. When feeling down or depressed I take a three day fig-fast, in three fig lunches. It's a sure-cure for the uglies and the munches, and maximally creative—you're sure to get hunches. Fast on lemonade all morning, and then have 5-10 figs for lunch, then fast to the next lunch. I love the fig-fast, for even dried figs are the fastest fruit cleanser, five times faster than a grape. Or use raisins (the grapecure) which are twice the quick-clean as a grape. Use these short fruit-fastarian vacations. When considering a complete fast you'll be relieved to remember our slogan "fig fast ok". This 24-hour fast followed by the fig eliminates all gut-residue seeping from the cells in that span of time. Since the gut reflects on the face in a fast, in a new role and face you've been cast. After three days of such reversal dieting, add cheese to again be frugi-fat-fastarian.

BE BEAUTY TO LOOK UP TO

To help sick humanity you must look like eternity. Wrong eating brings self-doubt and then God's help and promises are null--for there is no faith. The problem is always lost faith from befuddled mind and blood. God wants to save your associates by producing a masterpiece in you. That's why fasting is mentioned as often as prayer in the bible: Daily fasting and prayer defines the prosperous saint. Nothing will give you peace but the right diet for man combined with God's quick device of fasting for the few, His champions--that means you. And peace will mean prosperity. Are you in the problem or the only solution—to stop/postpone everything until you fast?

AGELESSNESS: SAINTS CHOOSE BEAUTY
Beauty is your Duty

Be ageless. You must, for the saints choose God's beauty—that's always the final reason to repent of "uglifying" sins. The reason you ate wrong was due to cultural hypnosis--glorifying carbs and damning fat.   Age is only one thing: morbid accumulation. Who could have known that you clean your veins through fat, unless schooled in metabolic (hormonal) sciences while being strong enough to discount cultural phobic mythology surrounding dietary fat? When combined with the fast the result is streamline and divine luster. Follow this plan and age signs will disappear and you'll die looking like a young child. Wrong foods will chemically reverse you to the other system as they are age-dependent: the older you are the more you'll look your age after eating them. if you aren't eating these false foods age will have little bearing on how you look and feel. All around we see premature aging because all around they're eating wrong.

With high-carb food everything ages: skeletal structure, skin system, facial structure, proportions, grace, alertness, posture, attitude (from "yes it can be done" to "no it can't—I'm over the hill"), hair, eyes, teeth, nails, and the way the feet and hands look (the ends show all). Since the same bloodstream furnishes every cell, iron red blood makes its mark as every pore takes on the same translucency. Once you see this and change your ways you'll take on the symbol of youth, innocence, the future and superior mind powers. You will no longer be held back by your own mood swings or compulsion to spend your life eating. Age will be irrelevant as in your elder years you'll still be the skinny shiny child. As a fat-fastarian you'll be a reflection of God made in his image, for "fat" is another word for "holy spirit" or the "annointing." Oils and fats--they conduct spirit and here they are the very things we've been told to stay away from. Now that you know what bad food does, just forgive yourself for eating it and start a brand new life.

FAT AND FASTING GO TOGETHER

Fat and fasting go together, simply because of the extreme appetite suppression a little fat creates. I would say fat defines this fast. The champion is a higher scientific spiritual artist who wishes to maximize the benefits of eating right. No matter what one's field he is sure of a high-yield. Mini-fasting will take you to your highest calling and every day will be a new adventure. If you're a writer, painter, musician or scientist it will catapult your talents up to the world. With each day digestion, assimilation and elimination moves while your fine talent improves. You'll find things are swinging in brand new grooves.

You'll go insane without fat on the brain. For in any field the social pressures remain. The fat-fast allows you to "get along" in the main. Miracles abound: as the fat smoothes your bearing you're fun to be around. Fat-happy and well-oiled neither the past nor petty people can clip, cut or   choke the creative coming into completion. The only way to overcome the brick wall and strut your stuff fast forward to the future is to collapse the past--which is just empty repetition of sin cycles and sick systems--and create a brand new reality without going anywhere. World travel can be tedious or terrible but creative mind travel is free and comfy in your own niche through the fast. What seems like nothing is actually everything, yet a free gift from God.

PENCIL-SHARP

Fatarian-fastarians are pencil-sharp and chisel-wedged because the face is an exact reflection, a diagnostic picture of the whole: When filled with carbs all interstices bloat up to resemble a white polar bear. When clean the puffy water-logged obstruction from insulin dissolves and one's features come "out" again. There is a vast difference between glucagons and insulin so the starchy vegan diet will not carve out or sculpt the interstices between bones and tendons to give the sharp look--the real features of the True Self. It is now fashionable to say "I am fruitarian" but when bulbous in feature because of the water-retention of insulin someone may ask "so what?" A bloated body is a sign of poisoning which constant insulin spike surely is. Look around--bloat is accepted as the way the human should look! Go to streamline: by denying hunger pains you are carving out another "chunk" from the gopher-like food face. So let the tummy burn and take great delight in it.   Get thin, for the skinny horse wins the race and the face.

With a little understanding fatarianism is in the back of everyone's mind--it is primordial, the carved look of shiny but soft jade. This recognition of "divine luster" will save lives. It is so primal: something they have never seen in this generation but will surely recognize. If you look too wide, irregular, lopsided or any other contrast from the "heighth-width index" of the fat-fasting hunter (the encephalized elongated head of a monarch) you're no evidence of the land of "milk and honey" but will be soon as you attract the money. One cannot lie about the highest! The correct curvature of the skull--the cranial index--should resemble an African child (with the energy on top-back of the head). When eating badly this will instantly be changed to the ordinary "adult" look of the white west created by carbs and the constant packing-away and wearing of everything we eat. But fat-fasting makes the switch, and fast.

HUNGER IS FROM EATING

Hunger is not dulled by eating for food only triggers more hunger. Before I learned this I was in a self-made jungle of fruit trees I couldn't escape. I finally saw I had to endure a little stomach pain, allow the encumbrance to dislodge and clean out and simply wait for hungry-free fasting bliss to return which it always did. The non-fasting fruitarian eats because he thinks he's hungry and he's hungry because he eats. When "fasting on high" even one grape can invite food demons in while just eating a little fat or continuing to fast would make them disappear, so persevere. Craving is just cleansing--endure the fires of frustration so that your conversion is true. Every yogi finds he must finally fast to complete his journey—it's a must opposing lust. Clean out the old life through this timeless rite of passage or continue to rust.

FROM SIN TO SYNCHRONICITY

Become a daily faster and you won't have to worry about anything anymore--it will all come in mass attractions to your unique self. You won't have to worry about the day, your agenda, who to call, how things will work out, how you look or whether you will succeed. Experienced fasters know that just by fasting everything works out on its own. It's an anointing that comes on a person--the spirit of fasting--that takes care of everything effortlessly with "holy spirit ease."   You can be struggling for months with a problem only to see it resolved instantly while fasting. It may be invisible now but it's all happening underground in a "fertile anarchy" as all atoms re-assemble into a new matrix--the new you.   Remember the slogan: "Indians don't work--they fast."

HOLY SPIRIT EASE

Become a faster and magic coincidences will follow you everywhere. As Jung said to his students "a scientist should never drink" as he would miss this fascinating synchronicity occurring only in the right-brain--which instantly turns off with compulsion, drink or insulin-elevation (constriction, bloat, hunger, hypertension, moods). Just eat fat and you'll look divine as you experience the world as God does: blissfully, for you're an oil "slick." Eat the icky concoctions and you'll look illogical since man's inventions make no sense to God's enzymes. Looking and feeling crazy you'll compensate due to lack of confidence through slips of the tongue and a dense muddy aura.

All bad habits cause anosignasia--loss of the right-brain's pattern recognition. Having lost the ability to recognize patterns in our lives we do stupid things in extreme tunnel-vision. In this state we are killing ourselves but can't see it. To get straight with food we must face the demons and stay conscious or they'll again drop unconscious while mindless eating ensues again. Your refusal to give into carb-cravings burns the split out. We go from timid conformity and covering tracks to one-pointed mind power. Whether rich or poor, male or female, young or old we now have the power of Queen Mother in the body politic. For this is a psychological diet par excellence—milk and honey reconstellates you back into your original condition or form. You now feel and think the way you were designed as a unique being with no more mistakes or bad acts--you are free to lead the way you're supposed to.

MAKING GOLD

People are debased through lawless and boundless body cravings. We must transform these instincts--make gold. The greatest people perform this alchemy to unify the conscious with the unconscious through the fastest way--fasting. Using the method of fat-fasting this daily mini-fasting life is simple. Why? Because the longer you adhere to this biochemically correct lifestyle the less appealing dietary indiscretion becomes.   When you're in the correct balance--not the culturally false idea of balance--you feel so good: mentally sharp, physically strong and emotionally stable.   But when you vary from this biochemical balance you feel so lousy that you ask yourself "why did I eat that?"

MAN HAS TWO SIDES

Man has two sides: persona (image) and shadow (dark instincts). Polite society may hide it but this split remains--though it falls unconscious, burns a hole and recycles life into a mundane blur.   To get to the miracles we must unify consciousness through facing and refusing the fires of desire. The frustration of desire then wipes out the compulsion and the bad memories feeding it. Denying this split rather than facing and resolving it keeps us split into two people: one "intending" to do right, the other obstinately doing wrong. Then the desire becomes a blind compulsion as he becomes its servant.

At lower vibrations there is no synchronicity, only split. When unified, energy is released and perception is opened. This released archetypal energy is the deepest and most profound and thus the most important to man. Refuse sin and watch major changes occur in miracle after miracle. The blood--what is in our blood--determines our miracle-level. When in a system where the only way to fit is to slip or split (as stereotypes are projected and one is pegged), fasting overcomes all. The alchemal fast will bring on the highest synchrony and an inversion of all systems: the top will become the bottom and the bottom the top.

TRANSFORMATION AND POP-LOCK

Hold fast with frustrations and soon you'll shoot to eternity. After refusing to give in to the fires of desire opposites unite, the split is gone and the experience is POP (instantaneous conversion) and LOCK (locked into a new dimension--there is no going back). When we fast on habit, frustration creates fire and then the psychic opening called aperture syndrome. This is an energetic theory: when energy is released it frees the mind of clutter--superfluity and excess and our true instincts (our genius) break from all culturally-imposed false instincts. In freeing the gold from the dross, the spirit imprisoned in matter, the result is refinement. We go from gross, unrefined and raw (the primitive addicted lower self) to refined, pure, dignified (the evolved True Self). Until then one is helplessly hooked to the distorted implants of other people—mostly about food—so endure for the sake of your brand new life: this will all be worth it and the sun will shine in the morning.

It's all just energy. The energy is invested in instincts. Caught in this stronghold we become lopsided, split and compulsive as this "shadow" drops unconscious. When we face the shadow (admitting we were sinners) and refuse to give in, we pop--and unite. The "pop" is the psychic opening that frees the spirit imprisoned in matter as we become true body mystics. If a big ego over-reaches itself it falls into hell for as weak kings conform to herds they degrade with them. But strong Kings with great longevity and lasting value transform their instincts--thus passing the test that brings their weaknesses and impurities to the surface. Are we really made of what we think (and boast) of?

ANYONE CAN EAT

Anyone can eat but are you strong enough to not eat? Humility precedes success so have the humility to say "I was powerlessly gripped by my shadow--my untransmuted instincts-- which I must now transform through self-denial." Sin sets in: someone can be a vibrant fastarian but then after nibbling on culture-food all the cravings and justifications come back. Suddenly he's surrounded by "good guys" who want the same and he's back in hell in drastic contrast to where he was. But because the frontal context never wants to blame the food the blame is shifted to outer events and other people.
It isn't easy to get back at this point--the now-bruised ego can't swallow pride that easily. One has relapsed into the same old cravings and the networks supporting them. In most cases one never gets back unless vain enough to desire God's beauty more than anything else--and this isn't vanity but the perennial desire of all the saints through time. When this poor relapsed soul is told about fat-fasting he is shocked: "that will never work and it will kill me." And so he is "just eating breakfast with friends." All is forgotten about the promises of the new life--he is now ordinary though popular. He can't wake up to free the spirit imprisoned in matter since the "matter" is delicious food acclaimed as healthy by culture, family, history, his cronies and the medical profession.

Freud said "we must not abandon discoveries simply to make them palatable" or culturally-acceptable. Where are the strong men and women who can keep to discovery despite the catastrophic collision with culture and the drastic daily discipline it takes to sustain it, or despite the rejection from family and friends when following it? Only a person who would rather have the character and looks of God: the ageless allure, the safety and protection, the quick wit and edification of mind and talents--rather than social approval and dulled-down deceitful and mundane "family love" of gorging and gathering as they gab. In short, the champions.

Free the spirit from matter. Making gold is not mere fasting but not doing a dead habit any more. Go beyond worrying and all that working for addictive foods to thinking about life and the quality of that life. See how little you can live on--the mini-fast with fat makes it simple as "pie." Fast and join the ranks of the timeless miraculous shining saints. Sacrifice and take the reward. The less you use the more God presents with presents. "I will increase as you decrease."

EAT WRONG, BACK IN BONDAGE

If you continue to play food-games with yourself, before long you're stuck in the swill with no exit. You never know when the bomb shall fall: when that terrible craving will hit like a demon sent from hell, an outside force over which you have no control. That is the effect of the wrong diet and of insulin. In its grasp untransmuted dead habits become possessive and the autonomisms begin: uncontrollable utterances and acts that can shame you for life. What do you care at this point? The insulin-run mood swings and irritability makes these things seem right at the time. You've lost the smooth fat consciousness, the even and poised bearing. A dead habit is psychosis--a complete loss of reality called addictive perception. Fat won't addict and you'll be eating less of it each day. But sugar and starch is fixed--ending in depression, fatigue, despair and eating more with time. Fast, or it's just another lost day compared to where you could be. Waste no more time in food-crime for on your consciousness it forms a slime.

FAST AFTER THE BINGE

You had a feast and now you're full. So what--just start now by looking forward and enjoying the fast. Just the mere decision to fast releases PHF--positive healing forces--that change perception and the body. No matter what you did, go from here and fast to forget the past.   All food tragedies can be the final lesson which will now stick. The greatest lesson I learned was the value of simplicity in foods to reduce craving and increase "found time" for other things. A complex food life of great variety is never satisfied and causes constant craving. We must see the energy waste of buying, procuring, fixing, eating, convalescing after and eliminating food. It just naturally attracts people on the same level who are also stuck in cement--carbs and the craving clan.

To eliminate the biggest addiction is the hurdle of one's life. It'll make you a king who can optimally enjoy life's lucid experiences when free of the eating game. Keep this slogan: "eating never makes me happy but fasting always does." "Eating never solves problems but makes them worse, fasting always finds solutions and clarifies all." It will put you on top for once and if you continue to live this way you'll stay on top.

RECYCLING OF ENERGY INTO CONVERSION

It's the biological instincts which become compulsive and must therefore be transformed, otherwise consciousness narrows and compulsivity throw one out of grace--while all his energy is recycled in outworn channels (patterns of addiction). This means trouble. The last tragedy brings so much stress that one finally "renunciates" and transforms his instincts into higher creative and expanded vision. This is the happiest day of his life having released the chains of misery and habit.   Until this transformation the high-life is blocked and life dulls into routine.   The compulsive eater beseeches and blames God: "When will my breakthrough come?" or "why have you forsaken me?" Only when he repents does his life finally change as he steps into a miraculous inner journey. The narrower the vision by compulsive actions the more autonomisms (disruptive uprushes from the unconscious) ruin his life. The devil made him do it? No, the complex processes and consequences of addiction made him do it. The robot circuitry is mixed up--the higher self being dead, the demon runs wild. He must transmute his lower instincts or the result is disaster. The red Indian is not lopsided: perfect on one side, bloated on the other showing disunity, duality, dichotomy. This is the look of the West and indicates flagged fascination with life: From one-pointed mental power the rod is cut in half and both sides dull to dim. Instead the beautiful shiny red Indian fasts and is unified with self God and nature--through a clean (glucagons-elevated, vessel-dilated cholesterol-burning) bloodstream.

REDSKINS UNITE!

Clean the body through fat and fasting and you become a redskin with iron-built blood. Eat culturally, you become puffy white. Indian's don't work they eat right then fast as everything comes to them. Fasting attracts prosperity--miraculously creative lucrative ideas and witty inventions. The "redskin" has cosmic understanding (the brain is being properly fueled with ketones), mystical knowledge, youth, beauty, creativity and an unfolding future. The "white" man in contrast shows only mental decay, material contamination (fat-storage), spiritual degeneration (too blocked up), age (dry skin and wrinkles), ugliness (it's the food not the genes) and all doors closed to further opportunity (no attraction).

BE A LEAN RACY GREYHOUND

Fast, the lymph cleans out and now you're red from iron and cleansed veins. Brush your skin and the white (glygogen) flakes off and you're no longer a flake. You still may have scaly hands but the cleansing process will in the end reach the ends. With the ends clean it's your end--completion gained and now success. You're now a lean, racy, long-legged and ornamental shiny greyhound: a silent mystery, a gentle world beauty, an avatar, a bright shining light to look up to, to model after. Now you the would-be hero becomes the magic shaman, the example of God's magic through his fat food which God specifically gave us to eat from the beginning of time. Fatarians like the beautiful Masai or Eskimos have no heart attacks or other diseases of modern civilization, all the while eating fat constantly and exclusively.

CLEANSING REACHES A HEAD

The cleansing process reaches a head like a dissolving sweat and fever. One day you're very sick as fat pockets dissolve and eliminate but the next day shows beauty and rapture from God's ingredients. Show neatness and aristocracy, without hypocrisy! With lymph cleansing everything puffs up around the mouth area with ugly lines. That is glycogen from carb coming out of the nasolabial folds seen in most low-fat dieters. Gravity pulls dense elements down--"turgidity"--and the ankles and calves swell. The arms resemble leprosy as the lymph cleans out. You thought that was just "aging" but the next day's elimination takes it all out forever--it will never be seen again unless you eat those starchy refined carbs again. We go from the worst to the best and that's our test--to not eat at temporary discouragement but instead proceed to the crest. Once you've hurt enough and still refused to eat God removes the test and gives the best.

TRIBULATION PRECEDES TRIUMPH
Endure the Cure Then View the Mirror

It was the most painful day of my life preceding the best day of my life. On this particular hellish day I had the occasion to describe the process in my journal:

"As the arms explode we see potential lymph cancer coming out--the cell-proliferation in the arteries from insulin. When the blood finally runs clean new protein/fat nutrients can now enter the cells of the arms becoming fresh new moisturized skin again. And the fat on the back of the arms--seen on all carb-addicts--will now go away with carb-cessation. The lymph fluid is very sticky as every pore is oozing with storage. With fasting it coagulates and comes to the surface in temporary itching lasting a day. As the blood runs clear its like a trillion lilies blooming, opening and awakening suddenly. One can feel the starchy substance coming out of the bloodstream and then running clear once more. The lymph running along the bloodstream functions to absorb up all toxicity from the blood, going up each arm, leg and the trunk. Even in the skinny it is clogged as seen in wrinkled arms and legs. New nourishment can never get to the cells to rebuild new tissue because of this. As the lymph drains one may become constipated as the sticky blood gum coagulates in the colon. While the sludge goes through the bloodstream you may feel very fatigued. Just sleep. On cleansing days you may feel and look your worst as the lymph drains out but the next day it's all eliminated and you go from worst you've ever been to the best."

FAT-FASTARIAN CORNUCOPIA

It is fat which cleans the veins. Fat elevates glucagons which is a pathway to the good eicosanoids which dilates airways and blood vessels, increases oxygen, enhances the immune system, prevents platelet aggregation and decreases cell proliferation (cancer). Insulin from starch and sugar constricts airways and vessels, decreases oxygen flow, suppresses the immune system, causes platelet aggregation and increases cell proliferation. Fat opens everything up, sugar closes it all down. The poor asthmatic can hardly breathe when eating sugar and starch, but if he takes some fat the airways open up to his great relief. What a shame the medical profession professes just the opposite, insisting people avoid the only cure!

Yes it's an amazing thing how the public has gotten rotten by seeing everything in reverse. There were no heart attacks in the nineteenth century though they ate many courses of fatty meats, butter, lard and cheese. They thought produce was an inferior food or just a table decoration. Just check out the thin cowboys in old photographs--they all resembled Paul Newman as they existed on eggs for breakfast and steak at night. Glucagons opens the vessels to keep the body streamlined. And thus fat-fasting is ageless cornucopia: Constriction shuts everything down and we feel miserable, but dilation delights in a glorious opening to a new life.

18

PALEO-FASTING

Fruit and Fat Means Never
Famished or Fatigued

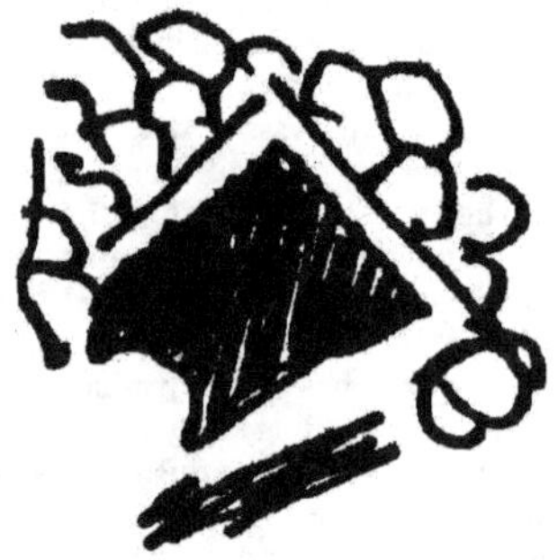

Modern science shows that man is like a CAT--he needs FAT and protein. Fat deprivation suppresses the immune system and brings other deficiency symptoms seen in people on raw, vegan or especially fruitarian diets. I learned this after twenty years of fruitarianism and the extreme craving for fat and protein which resulted in a failure to thrive (FTT) along with breathing and skin problems.   When I added fat my whole life changed and I was able to stay basically fruitarian with fasting each day: frugi-fat-fastarian.

BIG BRAIN TINY TUM

The gut-dense fatty food gave me a real feeling of lasting satisfaction that made day-fasting a breeze.   Fasting as a fruitarian made it very dull indeed--I was so malnourished I was fasting all the time anyway though eating constantly of the low-density, high-water and insulin-elevating sweet fruits. I was bloated, water-logged yet hungry thinking I was "spiritual" when actually I was "spacy" in a brain fog. Now I feel "bright" and paleoscientists have found that the gut-dense fatty foods release energy to the encephalization of the brain i.e. a bigger brain. The paleo foods like nuts or animal fat require much less for satiety and this releases digestive energy to the brain which enlarges thusly. Man's brain size decreased suddenly--de-encephalized--10000 years ago at the inception of agriculture which brought bigger starchier meals of grains and produce foods. With agriculture people grew fat and dumb!

The big paleo brain is linked to a small gut fed with small but potent foods which sustain him for long periods. Less food (i.e. bulk) increases brain size. Man has always been a hunter-gatherer eating fat and then fasting until the next kill: eating potent meals then not eating. Down with continuous fruit-eating and up with higher paleo-fasting bliss! There are some raw vegan "athlete guides" who insist their clients eat thousands of calories of fruit and vegetables and only ten percent fat. These poor athletes complain of constant hunger, craving, weakness, and being waterlogged from all the fruitless fruit and salad eating. It is ridiculous to fear fat for it would suffice and create energy for long periods without craving.

BLENDER AND LEMON-SQUEEZER

I feel so good on the higher paleo diet combined with daily fasting. I arise early before dawn and eat Greek Red Salad or doughless pizza with pineapple then fast to the next day. When I have avocados I make guacamole. There's no need for a juicer—just a blender and lemon-squeezer for light lemonaid. I like sweet juices but will avoid when I sense insulin-spike--to that puffy constricted feeling I say "take a hike". I'd keep nuts to chew and occasionally some raisins or a fig too. These foods are easy to store in organic bulk mail-order so no more running to the store. Get out of that old habit and reduce your foods to six—no more variety which only excites addiction and food-preoccupation. You want a new station and a millionaire occupation so go very light so God can strengthen your fight. He promises to increase as you decrease: jettison weight to float up like a kite.

TRAIL MIX FOR RECLUSES

The trail mix method is perfect for travelers or hermits. After I fat-fasted and stabilized I decided to lose my dependence completely on stores and fresh produce. I was just going to live on figs, raisins, nuts and cheese in one or at the most two mouse meals per day. I was never hungry and soared to the heights. Figs are powerhouses and the fastest cleansers of all the fruits. Raisons are the grapecure for cancer and easily stored while nuts are filled with vitaminerals, fiber and the paleo fat. For lacto-fruitarians cheese is much higher in protein and fat than meat and could be stored for six weeks in sealed packages. I found these six foods totally delicious and a wonderful balance to each other—sweet, sour, fatty fiber: lemonaid, black fruit, nuts and cheese. When I did shop I would buy lettuce, tomatoes, red bells and avocados have fresh lunches for two weeks until they ran out then the rest of the month trail mix. No need or urge to ever cook—why cook when you can have foods such as these whenever hungry, requiring so little due to their divine potency? Released from my lifelong food obsession I became continuously creative.

At last the inner journey and true independence could begin as the endless time-waste of daily meal planning and shopping was finally over.   The trail mix of black fruit and nuts made me feel very strong and happy for a long time and so trail mix is the greatest staple for the wilderness recluse and hermitage.   Juicy fruit has a short life so if one decides to fast it spoils. Solitude forbids running to the store to get juicy fruit and very few of us live on fruit farms. What is the answer? Nuts and dried fruit through the internet and storable for months. Dried fruit has all the vitarian (high vibrational) qualities without the insulin spike of juicy sweet fruit pervading the bloodstream.

HOME IS ALL

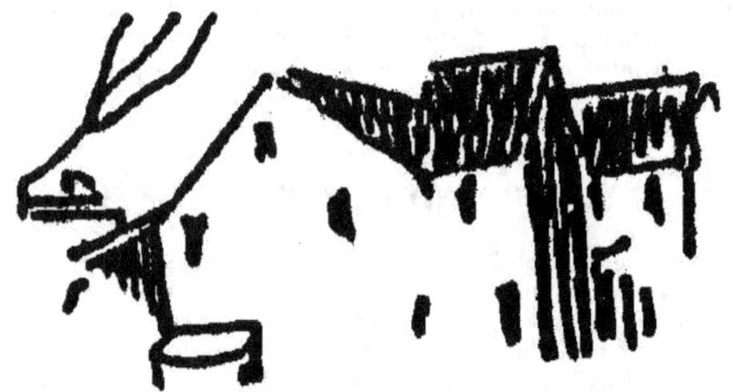

It gave me a real feeling of peace and security to live like this, perfectly set-up for months with a free-mind to daily fast and enjoy life without intrusion.   From these divine years I can truly say that there is no place like home! I have no desire to go to restaurants and eat around strangers or wonder about the cleanliness of the kitchen or cooks (are they kooks?). That's part of the paleo lesson—filling your home with staples of perfect foods lasting for months so you're truly free and never have to leave if you don't want to! I love my home, and losing one's home is one of the worst results of war.   Home is ALL. Home is our reality—it's where we don't have to adapt to other people.   More than anything else you must guard your home and let nothing in which is not good, perfect, divine and totally respectful of your authority. In this regard, be a caveman!

GOD'S FRUIT AND NUT TREES

Raisins and figs, nuts, cheese and olive oil: the perfect higher paleo diet for reclusion and home life of the spiritual man. Nuts, figs and raisins were the biblical desert and if you think about it they are basic. The triad of dried fruit, fat and fasting is a perfect set-up for long periods—even years--in nature independent of civilization.   Not being dependent on stores and being able to live solitude--even in Alaska or Siberia—while not being hurt by bad weather destroying the yield of fruit tress   gives a tremendous sense of satisfaction, freedom and security.   Having three months of food stored knowing it's the best makes you self-sufficient and in control of your own destiny. Man is a fat-frugivore, not a folivorous plant or leaf-eater so huge raw vegetable salads though tasty are not basic. Leave these things to the other animals with big guts to deal with all the bacterial putrefaction digestion these foods entail.   Just stick to the gut-dense foods and then fast to your delight without worry. Not until one has totally detached civilization and embarked on his inner journey in nature can he appreciate the non-dependence on civilized stores.   I didn't even require transportation anymore as my food was mailed to my door.

THE   HEAVENLY   TRIANGLE

When you need a cleanser what works better than raisins and figs? They eliminate (bind mucus) four times as fast as a juicy fruit like grapes and are also filled with iron and magnesium.   Then when you need a crunch or "bit" of protein and fat take a nut or two. They are so potent just a couple will suffice for long periods while keeping the gut flat—I like that. My favorite are the nuts highest in fat like macadamia (spread throughout the day they're a great fat-fast) but cashews are also delicious with raisins.   The cheese is much higher in fat and protein than meat and easily stored in sealed packages for four weeks. The cheese is a real "fauna-fat punch" that revivifies, for man needs fat and fauna-fat is pure paleo.   What a life—and what a way to restart the fast. In higher paleo-fasting each "meal" just starts the new fast so if you start a fast only to eat—so what? Just start it again. This is the highest guilt-free fail-free blend.

INSULIN: HEAD-ACHES AND HUNGER

Before the trail mix phase I had to heal my insulin resistance from twenty years of sweet-fruitarianism. After my overindulgence just a little sugar released a flood of insulin and all the maladies it creates (dry skin, craving, water retention, fatigue, constriction, irritability). But with fat and only frugal fruit I have no hunger or craving for I am balanced in the way man was designed from the beginning. As you proceed on this balanced diet you will find your mind ascending to higher creative levels and actually forget all about food. The Atkins dieter is into eating many meals and it gets crude. To me that misses the point because with fat you can forget eating and just create every moment—you transcend the physical altogether as new life ensues.

CHUNKY PASTY RELATIVES

With high-fat and low-carb glucagons signals the kidney to release salt and fluid, to the fat cells to burn stored fat for energy, to the liver to stop making cholesterol and triglycerides, and to the arteries to relax (dilate) and drop blood pressure. High insulin overwhelms glucagons so that we fatten and bloat up with water. In a miraculous way the fat-fast heals, regains balance and streamlines the body. The usual low-fat high-carb diet makes one chunky: as a fruitarian I was amazed to have a high cholesterol count though I never ate fat or protein.   Fructose raised insulin which cues the liver to produce cholesterol. What a paradox!

Hyperinsulinism is genetic. All my aunts and uncles were extremely obese and the "thrifty gene"--that which makes us pack on fat with very little bits of carbohydrate--was very evident. What that means is that all the nagging ailments from insulin--head-aches, irritability, hunger and craving, mood swings, depression and constriction--can occur with just one apple. I was so relieved to learn the perfect cure: fat for appetite-suppression, even moods and high energy. How very efficient: one fat meal allowing all other waking moments spent in fasting and creative action. My one year of fat-fasting amazed me in the way I suddenly felt and looked—from my mother's warning that' I'd end up like ancestors I was no longer spooked.

THE BODY IS ENDLESSLY MUTABLE

When fat/protein-needs were finally met the body-cravings instantly switched to include fruit and I had no adverse reactions from that point on. What this shows is that body heals through instinct, not by following "rules." The rules may apply at one time but are made inoperative at another. As immunity is boosted through fat and protein it's also suppressed through starch and sugar.   As our food history has varied so has our immunity which is endlessly mutable.   And thus the rules change for each phase of our life. Because of the present food fallacy of fat-phobia we have a generation of people with no or little immunity: the present epidemic of environmental illness (E.I.).   I live in the desert which is filled with E.I's escaping city chemicals. These are mostly post-hippies living on salads, pasta and other starches which only make them more sensitive. Every time the golf courses use pesticides they escape to another part of the desert, whereas due to my fat diet my immunity is improving daily and I hardly notice sprays.

For twenty years fruitarianism seemed so self-evident looking at food in a superficial light rather than the sophisticated understanding of how metabolism works. It's not that we are what we eat--but rather the metabolic processes that follow what we eat—whether insulin or glucagons is elevated determines our immunity and everything else.   It takes great mental strength to go against the fat-phobic masses who think produce and grains are best and fatty proteins are the worst--but you must. Just stick firmly to this regime and you'll see miraculous things happen to your body: extreme diminishment of size coupled with perfectly-formed muscles with minimal exercise.   The higher the fat-to-carbohydrate (ketotic) ratio the more ketosis--i.e. the more fat is burned and the less hunger. Lack of hunger combined with constant energy is a sign of ketosis. The brain and heart love to live off ketones, not glucose. During my day-fasting regime I felt best at   zero carb but when completely healed I could eat as many carbs as I wanted and feel great all through the daily 23-hour fast.

PALEO-SCIENCE

New paleoscience casts a whole new light on fruitarianism, rawfoodism and all vegan diets. The comparative ape studies which justified fruitarianism "because man is like an ape" are now in dispute for there are no fruitarian or vegan primates found in nature and captive primates on meatless diets had B-12 deficiency (beyondveg.com). Fruitarian tribes have never been found!   The truth is hunter tribes are healthier than farmers (storers of starch in silos) and fat-frugivores or -fasters are healthier than the fruitarian fantasy. What is the answer for someone who fears possible deficiency but is against eating meat?   Eat cheese, omelets and once in awhile a piece of fish. What a delicious dish as you proceed to perfect thinness (and anything else you wish).

I was seeking "purity" through fruitarianism. Having transcended this isolating ideology I opened up to the whole world through the original real diet for man which makes the body very happy.   As world trends go more towards the raw/fruitarian fear of mucus, protein, cholesterol, fat and cooking--all dissolves in the face of this new evidence. For the sake of your own health I hope you will transcend these idiotic ideologies based on philosophy rather than the fat needs of man.   If like most Americans you are stuck on produce and grains, a switch to fat and fasting will change your entire metabolism,   bloodstream, appearance and personality.   You will be and feel entirely different in a new revolution springing from complete hormonal change.   I can bet that all of your problems including the emotional have their basis in the high-carb diet including fruitarianism.

WISDOM SITS ON TINY BITS NOT FRUIT FITS

The benefits of fasting magnify after fat--suppressing all craving while releasing incredible energy for the day. This means no more highs and lows from hypoglycemia and carb-addiction, just a lovely even keel. I've known fruitarians who eat all day as much as they try not to. They're eating for satisfaction but after eating crates of such low-density foods any satisfaction is fleeting.   For those two years I found tiny potent HQ meals so much more efficient than all that water logging effect from produce. Original man ate like a cat--fatty protein was 95% of his diet.   He was just doing what came naturally in contrast to modern man who allows food fads to override his natural inclinations to eat luxurious deliciously satisfying fat. You must now refuse to doggedly determine daily foods through diet dogma which disregards the facts of evolution. To assist you here's the scoop on animal fat and protein: "fauna". To not give you the whole picture is to let you remain a blind beggar— you must open up to the whole reality from the beginning of time.

LARGE BRAIN SMALL GUT
Brain-Size Decrease with Grains

The paleodiet is around 55% protein, 30% fat and only 15% carb. The daily fast would be used in combination with paleo meals of fauna (cheese or raw eggs are fine), vegetables or fruit. Skeletal data shows that   homo sapiens have eaten meat for 2.5 million years but grains only 10,000. The human brain size decreased 11% in 35000 years and eight per-cent of this was in the last 10,000 years when farming began.   The introduction of grains prevented the brain from reaching complete genetic potential. In this time animal food dropped from 50% of the diet to 10% as grain came to substitute. This is the ratio of the modern diet and an explanation for the dumbed-down (though computer-literate) public.

The transition from hunting to farming had devastating health consequences across the world.   As the fossils show, the hunters had perfect health.   They were tall, lean, well-developed, strong with dense bones and sound teeth without decay. Less animal foods also means a consequent shortfall of preformed long-chain fatty acids: DHA, DTA, and AA are required for brain development and are much more plentiful in animal than plant foods. High animal: brain expansion, gut decrease. Agricultural: small brain, big gut. The bulk of brain decrease and gut-increase has occurred in these agricultural years.   The early increase in brain development is positively correlated with the level of animal food, a key component in Dietary Quality (DQ) that can never be filled by eating things like grains in its absence. Folivorous (leaves) diets correlate with small brains whereas fruit and animal foods with large brains. And thus man is and does best as a fat-frugivore.

BRAIN-GUT COMPETITION

Large brains may be the evolutionary result of selection favoring meat and high protein diet. Humans are distinct in the proportion of metabolic needs for the brain. Gut size is always associated with dietary quality so it must shrink to support encephalization (increased brain)-- suggesting high quality diet is associated with the large brain.   Only small bits of gut-dense fatty protein are required to satisfy hunger, burn fat and give the brain and heart the ketones needed for energy. This remarkable efficiency from small bits releases energy to the brain which then expands. The higher quality diet is more easily digested, liberating more energy and nutrients allowing encephalization.

FROM CARBS REFRAIN, THEN LARGE BRAIN

There is a limited energy budget and the brain and the gut compete for it. So much energy is required for brain growth that there is the potential brain size and an actual one. The large brain is always compensated for by decreased gut size--this doesn't come from huge vegetarian meals but tiny fat meals. The first increase of the brain was from the increase in animal foods. The second increase was from cooking since it reduced required digestive energy. Cooking neutralizes toxins and increases digestibility, freeing energy for the brain. All those raw vegetables are too "expensive" in energy terms. Raw is not law! Cooking is a high-tech way of "externalizing" the digestive process (reducing toxins, increasing digestibility) making digestion a metabolically less expensive activity for modern humans then for primates (beyondveg.com)

Here is Arello and Wheeler's finding as it was written in Current Anthropology in 1995: The higher quality diet brings increased energy which shoots to the brain as it enlarges it. Because it is reduced bulk it creates a smaller gut due to more rapid assimilation and this also releases more energy to the head. You increase dietary quality by increasing fatty (and also cooked) foods which enlarges the brain and decreases the gut. The modern (sweet/pasty) diet is more like half carb and fat and only 10% protein while the big brain diet is 55% protein and 30% fat and only 15% carbohydrate. Since fasting also encephalizes, fat-fasting is a "brainy" solution--a "longhead" marks the monarch.   This is so efficient for the champion life as opposed to continuous fruit-eating creating unstable blood sugar, fatigue, mood swings (often anger), acute sensitivity and the other characteristics of the fruitarian seeking "purity."

FAT FIGHTS FAT

The fat-fasting method can be described in two ways: (1) eating once daily followed by 24-hour fasting or (2) continuous fasting only punctuated with small bits of protein and fat—a piece of cheese, an egg, a nut (cheddar and macademia being the fattiest). I myself prefer the first method of eating only once in the day and blissfully flying off to a wonderful no-hunger fast for it is so much more spiritual to forget food altogether for 20+ hours a day. The daily "minifast" shows miracles abounding. It is so easily accomplished after a fatty meal and was nearly impossible existing only on fruit. Automatically your body begins to change: the gut used once a day shrivels to walnut-size. The sinuses open up as the brain awakes and expands. The lungs breath better than ever as glucagons dilates all airways. Suddenly you're a totally new human being and on every level the change is dramatic. Fat does not constrict and clog—on the contrary it dilates and releases.

WE NEED NOT LESS BUT *MORE* FAT, LIKE CATS

Human physiology shows we need more fat in our diets not less, and plant-based diets are lacking in sufficient fat and other cofactors such as B-12. Energy is stored much more efficiently as fat than as glycogen from carbs. Animals who get enough fat from veggies are less-active herbivores who need less efficient energy, but man is an omnivore who like the carnivore is far more active and needs a more efficient way of storing energy. Humans need fat for the skin to stay moist throughout life (vs. dryness and wrinkles), to stay warm (since we don't have fur) and for increased brain function due to higher intelligence. The synaptic connections in the brain are mostly fat and cannot function well in low fat diets. The studies of David Horrobin shows the improvement of emotional balance and brain function with high-fat diets. I myself can certainly attest to this—I was so up and down and at times so angry trying to live without fat. The slightest irritation would send me over a cliff. Coupled with this were constant cravings for meat—it was the fat I craved not the flesh. So important is fat to the human that the gut even tries to absorb preferentially what it needs through heme iron receptor sites (beyondveg.com).

THE HIGH-FAT MATRIX: A NEW LIGHT

The high-fat matrix forces us to see the world and diet in a whole new light. Things like eating a dozen raw egg yolks and then when cholesterol is checked it is normal! It is carbohydrate that evokes the liver and cells to create cholesterol, not fat--and glucagon which burns off all cholesterol. And as for things like asthma where physicians have always said to avoid fat, it is actually the case that fat dilates airways so that one can breathe. Fat releases constriction of the arteries, so while the fat-phobic masses see high-fat as death-threatening the more sophisticated understand this deeper metabolic science and scorn the superficial "you are what you eat" argument.   Energy is far more efficiently stored as fat and almost all cells can use fatty acids interchangeably with glucose for energy. The ability of cells to store carbs (in glycogen) is slight but 200 times more energy can be stored in fat than in carb which is used up in 48 hours   (after which all turns to fat-storage).   This immediate storage potential in fat means less or no fat-storage!

THE ABORIGINE STUDIES

The aborigines in Australia are a very interesting group in that they develop a high incidence of hyperinsulinemia and type II diabetes when exposed to an urbanized western diet. Like many Americans they are genetically predisposed to disorders like heart disease and diabetes and they develop them quickly when eating wrong, making them great candidates for the study of diet and hyperinsulinism. The urbanized aborigine subjects were consuming a Western diet: grains and beans, alcohol, dairy, sugar and cheap fatty meat. This diet was high in refined carb (40-50%) and fat (45%-50%) and relatively low in protein (10%).

Then they ate their original native diet of 70-75% protein, 25%-40% fat and carb only 5%. Insulin levels dropped by almost half and their health vastly improved--though they were getting much less exercise than in the city. This is exactly what anthropologists learned from mummy and skeletal data: the carb-restricted high-protein/fat diet brings optimal health, strong bones and teeth while the low-fat high carb diet shows the opposite along with all the degenerative diseases of civilization: cancer, heart disease, diabetes high blood-pressure and obesity.

GOOD   AND   BAD   EICOSANOIDS
Controlled through Diet

Let's understand the effect of the good eiconsanoids coming from fat vs. the bad eiconsanoids from sugar and starch. As Sears says in The Zone: "you can view eicosanoids as the biological glue that holds the human body together--the most powerful agents known to man yet totally controlled by the diet." The good eiconsanoids are the very definition of optimal health. When they're balanced the skin glows and the system hums in perfect health. When the wrong ones are evoked the result is aging dry skin, arthritic aches and pains, blood clots, arterial constriction, asthma and heart disease.

Good Eicosanoids: From fat, glucagons is elevated and the result is: dilated airways, increased oxygen, vasodilation, immune enhancement, decreased inflammation, decreased pain, increased endurance, the prevention of platelet aggregation and decreased cell proliferation. Bad Eicosanoids: From starch and sugar insulin is elevated and the result is: constricted airways, decreased oxygen flow, vasoconstriction, immune suppression, increased inflammation, increased pain, decreased endurance, platelet aggregation and increased cell proliferation.

What an incredible revelation to the fat-phobic masses: the fat actually dilates (opens) the veins and airways so that the asthmatic can breathe. It decreases the platelet aggregation that constricts arteries and the cell proliferation which is cancer. What an amazing way to recover: a wonderful fat-fasting vacation where things like rashes, asthmas and other nagging ailments completely disappear. Try the fat-fast for four days: just eat high-fat and protein foods keeping carbs beneath 30. If there is no weight loss keep them under 15. If still fat go zero-carb for awhile and keep to the fast:

Carbs: Asparagus (6) 3, Broccoli (cup) 8, Cabbage (cup) 8, Cauliflower (cup) 5, Celery (3 pc) 4, Cucumber (6 slices) 2, Green beans (cup) 6, Lettuce ((1/2 head) 6, Mushrooms (cup) 4, Onions (1/2 cup) 6, Pepper 6, Radishes (4) 1, Spinach (cup) 8, Tomato (1) 4, Zucchini (cup) 5, Avocado 9, Lemon 6, Olive (10) 1, Peach 10, Plum 9, Raspberries (cup) 9, Strawberries (cup) 7, Apple 18, Pear 18.

Everything from sagging wrinkled skin to paranoid mood swings will disappear after adding fat to the fruit diet. After years of vegan vulnerability you must drastically boost immunity or die. The daily meal and then daily fasting will create such a sudden transformation and rejuvenation you'll want to shout and tell the world.   I could not believe it as I finally had the "look", the feel, the experience I was seeking (to no avail) through fruitarianism.

ONE MEAL A DAY IS THE MINI-FAST
So just eat it first--no need to fear it.

ONE MEAL is sufficient for many people and they can immediately enjoy the benefits of the mini-fast of 22 hours daily. This meal can be as large or small as you please—but I guarantee it will make the fast happy, satisfied and free.   The daily evacuation of the one meal (esp. if followed by a few nuts) is an amazing benefit of the higher paleo diet. If you're coming out of a deranged food history you'll feel good on cooked vegetables and even spuds for the transition.   Once properly detoxed you may eat all raw fruit, fat and then fast contentedly or you may enjoy starches with it—after all most of the world and every continent lives on starches with God's plants and our pet cow/goat's raw milk, cheese, cream and butter for our French dishes that bring maximum satiety for the happy days for the rest of our satisfied and healthy life. After I reached my target weight of 100 lbs (like a jockey, ecto-ecto) I can enjoy all foods including starches for my break-fast every morning. Being Scotch my family and childhood were BIG ON BUTTER and they were bone thin. I love baked potatoes with butter and sour cream and doughy pizzas with extra cheese and whatever else I want—and I stay gaunt showing style and living in grace.

God doesn't want you scared like this. He doesn't want you thinking of the morbid past so much either sis.

19

RAMADAN FASTING

Sun meals and Arabian nights:
Eat dark, Fast days.

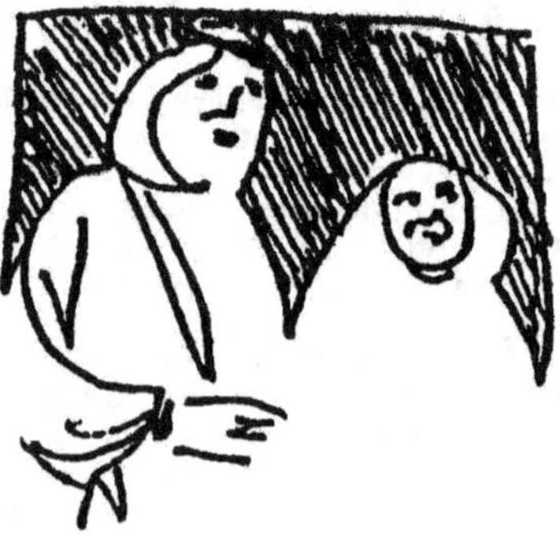

The Ramadan Fast is eating before dawn and after dusk—fasting during daylight hours. We Scotch love our big breakfasts as the most important meal of the day. I was always told it wouldn't matter if I ate again—I'll say it matters if you do! Being such an early-riser my fasting life is usually from breakfast-to-breakfast. I love Ramadan Fasting of eating before dawn and at night nothing or just a few nuts. Most Muslims eat far more for the nightly feast but I recommend keeping the nightly meal very slight for the sake of human growth hormone which perfects the engine at night if fasting. I love dividing the day into bipolar opposites day and night. The fast is for days to look your best, trigger your inspiration, illuminate your work and power in public. Eat only in dark--become a secret society as the king is never seen eating but maintains highest energy all day.

Fasting is mentioned in the Bible as often as prayer yet few Christians use it consistently as a rewarded routine. Not so in days of old when fasting was taken so seriously as a means of overcoming enemies, receiving God's guidance, clearing out physical ailments, eliminating demons, healing the sick and doing God's work under the anointing---His tangible spirit making burdensome work a breeze. Fasting works and it's rewarded by God every time so it should be done consistently and with great deliberation. It should be our trump card, our ace-in-the-hole when all else fails. It should be looked forward to with great expectancy and glee as a wonderful gift from God to enjoy and use as a fail-free device to receive His Power. For the faster all problems dissolve.

Fasting should be taught to our children more than anything else as the way to control appetites and improve character--as it has been passed on to one billion Muslims across the world. Ramadan is the month-long Sacred Fast of Islam. Fasting is one of the major pillars of Islam--not just another incidental bit of ignored law. To get to God's infinite power we must fast and without it we simply won't experience His bountiful blessings and promises. Learning of Ramadan was the beginning of my consistent fasting life every day after breakfast. Only by stepping out of my usual matrix and investigating another lifestyle could I really see the sacred fast for all the beauty and bounty it brings. As you fast think only of God--let Him pour his wisdom into you. Afflict (deny) self to get to His mighty power. Fast today and miracles will flow your way.

EAT   THE   SUN

Ramadan is no eating during daylight hours--we "eat the sun". During the day we fast and at night we eat--night and day are as different as black and white. Arabian (desert) nights, how you shine in blue and purple so different from bright days of yellow and gold! I have always enjoyed fasting this way long before I knew anything about Ramadan for I live in a hot desert like Arabia where day and night are like two different worlds. There are two different sets of wildlife: those who arise at day and those coming out at night. Everything is in these same two sets--dark and light. When not given denser food during daylight hours the fasting body automatically re-adapts to grasping all nutrition from higher sources--the sun and air is our "light lunch". How easy—you start the fast full, then enjoy the day with maximum energy as digestive energy is transmuted into creative action without lull! Devoid of food the days are more fun and miraculous than the nights for we rise to far higher pleasures. Since food is usually the biggest distraction its deletion from our thought life brings an explosion of new openings and vistas of thought during daylight hours and then at night the festivities begin, a salute to the achievement of the day. The days are totally creative as the glorious light shines on our work and brings it to completion. The desert is such a special place to prove this out.

PREDAWN   MEAL: THE   SUHOOR

I have always enjoyed a predawn meal (the Arabian name is "suhoor") followed by a fasting day feeling so exuberant living off this highest invisible nutrition then taking a siesta or just meditating in the afternoon fasting state. Then when dusk falls it is an entirely different night adventure and the post-dusk meal called "iftar" which for me is a few raisins, nuts or nothing. This type of Ramadan day always ends in cozy deep sleep and waking up so refreshed. Learning about Ramadan fastomg taught me how to appreciate more of God in this day-process thinking of Him constantly. It cast a much more serious—edifying--light on the fast, for beyond better health you'll also be rid of various appetites bringing your downfall. Self-control over the instincts and other troublesome traits builds great character. Your talents can really take you places but only your fast-built character will keep you there.

Ramadan fasting is difficult if eating an insulin-elevating breakfast. Starch, sugar or fruit will catalyze your appetite to start the day in hunger. This is shooting yourself in the foot before you even run the race! Elevate glucagons through fat and you'll start the fast in ketosis in top speed and exhilaration. You'll get a head start if you eat to ketosis then fast to championship--don't ever forget that sugar and starch (and for a few of you even fruit) is your enemy. As far as sugar is concerned you may never retrieve normalcy but fortunately I did, for I love fruit. Now I enjoy melted cheese with garlic and cashews with pineapple on the side. This is so satisfying there is no hunger for 24 hours or more.   During my year of fat-fasting I had an early cheese omelet and knew I wouldn't be hungry again and could just enjoy the day--knowing I looked and operated at my best. Having eaten fat I was a ready rocket but with sugar and starch I was a dead log and the fast was miserable.

I've gotten so into the fasting part of the day that the suhoor meal is increasingly just a mainstay--a way to sustain the fast. Just watch what happens as the food obsession is replaced by higher creative thoughts. Knowing you won't be eating during the day, a torrent of creative action is released. You'll see that despite your age you're a dynamo, like creativity and problem-solving never ceased! You will love how you feel, how things look, how music sounds, how vital you are. The compulsion to eat in order to deal with deep gutsy issues will now be dissolved as you face them instead to be replaced by a new joy of living. You'll see why a book on psychology should contain so much on fasting—the over-comer's device of victory and healthy-mindedness.

HOLY SPIRIT EASE--IT'S A BREEZE

Fasting is the fastest way to build great character and it's taught to very Muslim child as a major pillar of life. I have a saying about success: whatever the burdensome work postpone it until tomorrow and just fast today. When you wake up the irksome activity will be a snap! We should fast for our success which occurs via revelation, separation and reconnection: Since all disease is obstruction our recovery occurs by elimination. Once having cleared the way it comes in by attraction alone.

Whenever I'm feeling timid, uncertain, confused or creatively dry I hang my burdens needs and hopes on the fast to fix it. If there is fear, the fast removes it. If there is doubt the fast solves it. If there is dejection the hole inside is filled by the Creator himself while on the fast. With each day you'll be more sure of life itself. As we age do our powers wane? Not ever on the fast as we have all the power of our maker at our disposal.   The fail-safe fast is free so let it be your front. Just be silent as all the power of God swoops down to fill the gaps--it ends energy saps and spiritual lapse.

NIGHT VS. DAY

I love day fasting: getting up while it's still dark, feeling so good because of the previous day's fast, preparing the predawn meal and thanking God for both this and the new day.

This predawn meal is blessed and we should gratefully eat it in silence and feel renewed as we prepare for the day that lies ahead. What a wonderful way to start the blessed day--so different from the night. In a fasting state this day brings numerous blessings and lessons so we should ready ourselves in great anticipation.

What I love about the Ramadan fast is how it leaves you in a continuous state of readiness for anything during the day. No one should ever see you eating! With the rest of the world energetically down in the gut during business hours and you in the head fasting with angels--who will win? You will. With the day free of this absorbing compulsive activity miracles are now attracted in. It's amazing what happens when you "leave a space." Depending on how voluminous an energy-user your eating life was, this now-empty space will instantly transform your life--the more doors closed the more doors opened. Fast, wait on God and be ready for miracles. There's a champion aura to a faster so during business hours you win. Do it every single day of your life: stay fit, trim and alert--be ageless and achieve your goals.   You're achieving via the most ancient method given to man by God, so congratulations--you're now way ahead of your fellow man in a very competitive world. It's a paradox--the way you get to total power is to humble yourself like this for the ego wants to eat. To deny that grasping tiger is to humbly get the power of the almighty instead.

LIGHT   LUNCH

God divided the day from the night--and this light will be your lunch.   To God one day is like a thousand years and that measures your great reward. Great anticipation fills your soul--another day is a millennium of fasting miracles! This becomes more evident each and every time you do it so the early meal of "figs or fat" sets the stage.   Pray before the meal and thank God for the victory which lies ahead. Increasingly I appreciate day vs. night from the duality of my own desert experience. When one is depressed during the day instant relief is gained by saying "ah but soon night will fall and all will change." Depressed at night? Just say "Ah but soon it's another day and all will be different." That is how I view fasting vs. eating as the reversals bring continuous appreciations of something new.

Fasting eliminates impurities while cleansing the entire digestive track. You cannot imagine how perfectly digestion/assimilation/elimination works after a period of fasting—just one or two meals skipped. When people hear the word "fast" they panic as it congers up a long period. But Ramadan fasting is just seven lunches missed a week, while worlds of healing are accomplished in just one day. What great and mighty benefits: not only healing but exhilarating energy and inspiration—you should view this as your greatest accomplishment separating you from the world of taste-trippers at the mercy of food lusts! You'll so fall in love with mini-fasting you'll begin to do it consistently just because of how you feel the next day. It's like the housewife who cleans house simply because of how she feels afterwards, not because she "should."

Waiting to eat until night makes that final reward—iftar--a real celebration of victory, a well-deserved festivity of laughter and happiness. For a day in fasting is a great investment in the storage house of blessings for health, wealth and favor with man. When your children successfully fast one day be sure to reward them with great admiration at night--get it etched in their brain and they will always return to it with trouble, ill-health or the need for answers.

FOUND TIME: YOU'RE GETTING BETTER

As a Daily Fastarian one loses all fear of time passing by so fast (i.e. getting older) for with each day and hour he is getting better with more beauty. God says "fast and pray daily" and this is the way to do it--each and every special unique day. It's an upside-down kingdom in which one starts the fast with a feast. God is good--he's not a legalist who says "that's no way to fast--you must suffer." Oh you may suffer as hunger seeps in a little later but the more you afflict self the more you get to God's power. Self-affliction through fasting or the dissolving of ego is the main way to crush your feeble ego to get to the power of it all.

This generation is Dionysian, into pleasure-seeking. Many Christians agree with the necessity of prayer but balk at "fasting" though it is mentioned so many times in the Bible. The result of fasting is humility which always precedes success. Pride (self-indulgence) precedes defeat while humility through fasting precedes triumph.   The Bible says "There are some sins that only go out through prayer and fasting."   Perhaps only when used as a last resort will you truly learn its great power.

DAY FASTING BRINGS ORDER

The decision to fast daily brought tremendous order into my life. The mere setting up of the new matrix--involving food, a major part of life--kicked my whole day into new productive routine. With all daily food thoughts gone a tidal wave of creative energy was released. A fast? No sweat--for I can eat tonight.   Had I told myself "I can eat in thirty days" I might not be so happy. If someone wants to fast that way let them do it.   But daily fasting as a permanent plan can accomplish just as much while maximizing the daylight hours into productive activity and glorifying the night as a wonderful reward. This is optimal satisfaction and joy for the whole 24 hour cycle.   Arabian nights and a day of miracles occurs as man's major addiction and obstruction—food--is dissolved. This creates an empty space and a vacuum of attraction called pneumaticity in which the new life is "sucked in."

The two-speed matrix reviving life is feast vs. fast. Even if you eat the best food on earth you still need both. The feast celebrates the bounty brought on from the fast. The fast brings on the prosperity needed to cash-out the feast. It makes each and every DAY so special. As you fast with me you can know we are on the same spiritual wavelength--a world community of day-fasters. Think of the global telepathy that goes on between believing fasters! Fasting, like one good book can change things suddenly.

FASTING   CREATES   THE   FUTURE
Stop Procrastination

The brain can't handle two disparate thoughts simultaneously: negative and positive. Food can be so negative as a severe procrastination to fail--a way to block anxiety while going nowhere or getting worse! But the fast is a way to create the future as co-creators with God: having afflicted Self we instantly step into His power. The Self erased, the infinite power of God swoops down to take us off to the Great Destiny He has planned--our Highest Calling. Fasting gets the vessel into perfect shape to be ready for the camera, to show God to the masses! Your face carved on a coin, you become the eternal self God designed, the blueprint destiny: God's child, His peculiar delight and brilliant shining witness, not a blurred indistinct representative of the mass. Become unique through the fast. Through Ramadan you'll look superb and show the world fasting is where it's at. Let us share this day, every shimmering moment a divine witness to God. I'll be thinking of you in all our found time in this day, the only day.

20

BUDDHA FASTING
Afternoons with God

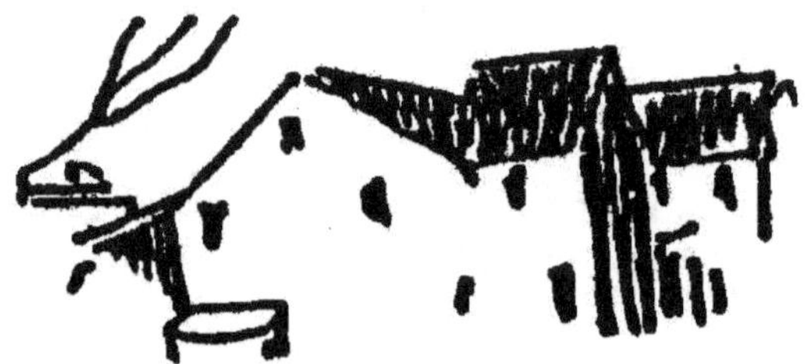

You've had your food quota by noon or maybe you feasted for breakfast. You can still fast the Buddha way which is not eating past noon. Just this method alone can heal so many diseases, for fasting from noon to the next morning is 20 hours. Done daily the healing benefits are cumulative.   The afternoon becomes a blissful digestive experience in sun or siesta, completely available for contemplation, study and prayer. This mental availability is what sets off the creative process both in the afternoon and especially the next morning. God rewards these partial fasts!

The Buddha fast really splits the day in two: morning for business, work, errands and the afternoon for quieter facets of life—contemplation, study, siesta, walking or correspondence. The morning fast is not unbearable as the mid-day meal approaches, then after we delight in a slow luxurious meal it is easy to make it through the afternoon and evening since the fatty lunch is so appetite-suppressing and satisfying. Then at night we're already in a cleansing state and the afternoon fast puts us in solid ketosis in preparation for comfy sleep and cleansing. Eating at night before bed is not smart as it's when nature cleans, so help it along by just skipping dinner to elevate this cleansing/perfecting/youthifying HGH—Human Growth Hormone. It only perfects while fasting.

Before noon I'll have figs then fats. The fat always dilates and opens everything up while streamlining the body.   The more fat-to-carb the better for energy fat-burning appetite-suppression and that wonderful cozy consciousness that comes from neolithic eating.   This way the afternoon begins with glucagons going into ketosis and a wonderful frame of mind which is so balanced and soothed.

BUDDHIST MONASTERIES FAST PAST NOON

The Buddha plan is the most popular fast and probably the easiest.   It's called the Buddha fast because it's the routine adopted in most Buddhist monasteries: arise very early in the morning (between 3-4a.m.) for prayer and meditation. Finish the main meal by noon followed by the afternoon's fast of more prayer and contemplation.   As Ben Franklin said "lunch with little, sup with less, better yet go to be supper-less." The first time I did it as a teen-ager I could not believe how exuberant I felt the next morning--it was a drastic change just by skipping dinner. I did it because I felt stuffed and fat but after just one fast I lost all that and more before the fat cycle began.

AFTERNOON

We've done our work, we've been rewarded with lunch now we're being inspired by fasting--i.e. keeping energy in the head rather than the gut. The afternoons will become your favorite time--in silence. This silent time brings found time for a multiplicity of other far more rewarding things. Fasting is always rewarded and it will bring you joy, extreme self-esteem, confidence and a real sense of superiority as a glorified child of God.

It's great to divide the day this way for anything bringing structure and routine increases productivity. I write in the mornings but the afternoons are the most productive relaxing into inspiration. Leaving it open this way readies the mind to receive God's words of instruction each and every peaceful afternoon. One should take this very seriously as a fast--20 hours daily from noon to 8 a.m. is a lot of fasting and healing. Yet it's so simple--a hunger-free afternoon: at night feeling so achieved and the tail-end when hunger may arise you're sleeping soundly.

The fatty paleo lunch will so change your consciousness. Whatever your emotional-mental problems were in the carb-laden fruit or starchy vegan diet they will all disappear now, setting your metabolism up in the opposite way--the way most beneficial for man, the way he was designed to eat. Like a cat, man needs fat. You'll be surprised as ailments disappear, as so many came from your carb-addiction creating hypertension, diabetes, coronary heart disease and simultaneous obesity. What a life--even now I notice that with too much fruit the skin gets dry and itchy but when again eating fat it soothes and revives into moistness again. It's a very "altogether" feeling with the fat which   is the most delicious food but has the additional pleasure of how you're going to feel afterwards.   Soon you'll see old habits dissolve and you'll be in a much happier state of mind.   Since the head and heart loves fatty protein (living off ketones) we now feel so much joy that old habits to avoid anxiety lose priority and then drop off completely.

MAN NEEDS FAT AND PROTEIN

Man needs fat and protein--that does not change. You say protein creates mucus? Listen up: the devastation that comes from (1) too much carb and constant insulin elevation together with (2) too little fat and protein is far greater than the problem of mucus and other by-products of protein digestion. The immune system is enhanced with fat and protein and suppressed by starch and sugar. Although nuts do well for fat and protein most people find they need fauna and any resulting mucus is eliminated through daily fasting and fruit. There are times when fauna-fat completely repairs and "fixes" things—an immediate streamlining, dilation and release of water retention takes place.

There is so much confusion in diet science right now. Due to the influence of Ehretism if you feel bad   they say you must have eaten something good   which brought on a cleansing crisis. If you feel good they say you must have eaten something bad   to stop cleansing. If any of this is true—why not use daily fasting as a way to offset problems and make things right? The gut-dense foods like cheese and nuts require so little to suffice it's amazingly efficient.

HUGE VEGAN SALADS OR PIECE OF CHEESE?
Raw is *Not* Law

And what of the huge salads people are eating--the predominance of plants and leaves? Man is not a folivore (plant or leaf-eater) as this requires a big gut for bacterial putrefaction. Beyond that some of us have so ruined our metabolisms via overindulgence in fruit (sweets) that these plant foods are really nearly impossible to digest--except when cooked--and the energy expenditure is far too burdensome until metabolic balance is restored.

For many of us years of "fruitless fruitarianism" brought us "mal-absorption syndrome" where we'd lost our assimilative capacity—the food just sits there and goes through unchanged. So is "raw" really "law"?   What a relief it is to leave the mass "raw" ideology behind, use what works in the interim then end mostly raw in the fat-frugivorous scheme while eating cooked at times. Relax and realize that diet dogma kills! There's no more blissful state than being on the evolutionary diet for man through ketosis--and many vegan foods may kick us out of it.

DETOX VS. EVOLUTIONARY MATRIX

What man has adapted to is the point. As a fruitarian I thought I was cleansing but I was filled with fat and water pockets from constant insulin elevation. The water was rapidly relieved with glucagons and I couldn't believe the relief with fats as a predominant part of the diet. You must start slowly now and experiment in the main fatty meal.   With each day you'll be stronger and your fat intake greater without a reaction. The total load on the immune system will be low (from fasting all day) so each day you will tolerate more.

Paleo science shows we need animal protein and the B-12 deficiencies of long-term fruitarians are usually the case not the exception (beyondveg.com). I did indeed feel a lot better during my "cheese omelet phase" after two decades of sweet fruit only.   For some of you the only fauna you can tolerate may be caviar!   Once you find the one thing that works--though all else may fail--just stick to that when you need a protein lift. Since it was protein malnourishment which suppressed your immune system you'll soon gain more latitude with food. Remember fat and protein strengthen immunity and grains ruin it (grain damage) so in a short time you can eat more variety. Via fat and protein the system is oiled until it glows so smooth--the look, the feel, the experience of living off the fat of the land--make it glow to show for dough! Then fast: return to perfection in total satisfaction.

If your a happy fruitarian that's great. You haven't reached the point of deficiency-burnout. But for those of you who are tired of the constant cravings (for what you instinctively want but deny) and the fatigue this section is for you. Until stable elevated insulin made me so restless with insomnia, emotional turmoil and flip-flops, water retention, depression, constriction, hypertension and dry skin problems. High-fat and protein eradicated the aged hanging skin ("scrawniness") by giving it glow and structure while it brought even-ness to emotions and energy. It erased all cravings, the biggest distraction contributing to failure to thrive. By keeping insulin low I became a different person for one year and through fasting I achieved.   I wanted glucagons to rule my castle not this temporary neurosis coming from elevated insulin in a person with IR.

LISTEN TO NO ONE

It's amazing how the world tries to cajole you to eat sugar (and starch) just when you decide to give them up, or tells you not to eat fat—most of the world is against fat! It takes a very strong mind to go against an upside down backwards world which calls evil good and good evil! Can't anyone think deep (i.e. metabolically) anymore? Must we stay so silly and superficial to blame the usual suspect "fat" for everything? Non-fructose sugar is the culprit and problem (along with starch which turns to it) and a deliciously fatty diet without refined sugar and starch is the answer. Most people fall in with the majority view which is fat-phobic and few understand metabolism--so the first step in maintaining your joy and slimness is to ignore the world of gainsayers. They're all out there so just be ready!

It's amazing how people will learn and accept hard facts and even understand the complex mechanisms of metabolism regarding insulin vs. glucagons but when they crave starch or sugar out the window it goes ("fruit is ok", "rice is ok because the Orientals eat it", beans are ok because Cosmopolitan said so" etc). Or they'll chime in with those calling the ketogenic diet "lost balance." But it was the past which was off-balance so now we must compensate by being "off-balanced" the opposite way. The present checks the past and this is balance. Once healed you take on the truly balanced diet of fruit and fat.

GET THE SHINE, THEN GOD WILL SHINE
God is the Only Source—Let Him be Your Course

We must find the fine line between shine and swell. The HQ (i.e. calorie-dense) higher quality fat foods like cheese and nuts can swell you up with overindulgence so you must respect it--find the line and keep to that, there's the shine.   Never overeat the HQ for the whole point is its potency in small bites but toxicity when overdone. Respect the greatest then never overdo it. Then having oiled the engine, fast all afternoon.   Get into it---notice how the inspirations flow and keep a journal of all the many miracles. The more you do it the more you'll love it.   The bonus is how you'll start the day tomorrow morning—wow! On the Buddha post-noon fast everything you do today is for how you're going to feel tomorrow.

Do you ever feel discouraged about your work or money? I know that especially with writing the remuneration is dubious and unstable at best. Always recite when down: "God is the only source!" Knowing that, all you must do is please God who will justify and bring out your work. No more self-promotion, racing around or feeling powerless in this competitive computer world. Just please God, not some clod, and all will come out right with you on top. What a relief stopping the biggest energy thief. He has a plan and you are part of that destiny and purpose which awaits—so just fast and continue to wait for that big future span. We fasters are a world clan much bigger than our problems which the divine fast is higher than! Soon you'll be winning for the way you please God is through sacrifice—fasting, giving and no more sinning. Now release your anxieties into joy ever-grinning.

BRIGHT WITH HOPE AND PROMISE

How I love the balmy-breezy afternoons which are so spiritual when fasting. I like walking all afternoon in nature with the dogs and desert angels. Then I come into study, contemplate, do yoga or just ponder while looking out the window to the mountain vistas. What a happy reverie! So much underground mental work is being done in the afternoon because you're in the relaxed right-brain mode. Insights won't arise with stress but only in leisure. True Genius is simply someone who knows the value of leisure for without it he stays frustrated, dry and third-rate. But fasting ensures that the fertile anarchy of the underground work brings maximum creative action the next morning—with success you have a date. Whatever your worry or work just fast and cast your care on God for tomorrow, for the fast He designed for man will work--for health, wealth and svelte.

MOST WILL GO BUDDHA-FASTING

I predict most will choose the Buddha fast for it's the easiest and it fits well into society. You can always "do lunch" or even early dinner and still be a daily fastarian. Perhaps many of you are already doing it but knowing the value of the matrix will keep you firmly in place--for it's the daily doing of it that brings eventual perfection and disease-free (fat-free, age-free) bliss. Think: "This whole afternoon and evening is mine, not the food-demons." This is always the highest destiny--the non-flesh, non-obsessed times with God and just knowing this opens you to infinite directions with a feeling of achievement, pleasure and hope. You now have so much reason to hope, for the exclusion of food for a good part of the day is so uplifting, enlightening, elevating and edifying. It will exhilarate you releasing so much energy and time normally tied up in food. This will change the whole consciousness of the afternoon and open up new avenues normally closed.

CUTTING IT OFF SAVES MONEY

Cutting it off at noon saves so much money. It's one meal rather than two so if you're now spending $300 for food now it's $150 or less for now as you have learned self-discipline and become healthier each day you order your food preferences rightly, eliminating "binge food" or other useless items. Now food-confusion is dissolved and all falls naturally into a new matrix. You know exactly what to buy for just the MMM: main mid-day meal. An afternoon eater is a promiscuous eater eating whatever his afternoon hypoglycemic carb-addicted taste buds dictate to him he "should" eat. But you with total self-mastery have deleted this phenomenal food waste so your bill may even be one-third of what it was.

STRENGTH

You say your strong? Let's see how strong you are--fast. Are you mentally strong enough to go against the fat-phobic carb-loving masses? Can you withstand the fruit- and fast-fears of the increasing mass of Atkins dieters or the medical dogma? And against those doctors-- still in the majority--who in the face of overwhelming new evidence on the side of fat still maintain you should live on high-carb low-fat diet? Do you realize what a dangerous concept that is?

The result is millions of unhappy people depriving themselves of what they need and urgently desire but deny, just to "go along" or "get along" with the majority or the neighbors. Atkins comments on how many people say they loved the first two weeks of the fatty low-carb diet, that they were happier and more satisfied than they've every been. When asked why they went off the diet they said "my neighbors didn't agree with it." When will people give up on the obvious and see beneath? To the mentally flimsy: you must question all that you've been told and once having learned all the facts stick firm against the ever-changing tides of public opinion which is usually nonsense.

WATCH SELF-WILL—IT TAKES YOU TO SWILL

Are you strong enough to not eat when you want to eat? That shows strength. The wishy-washy make resolutions--they intend--but at the first craving the ego bristles up and says "forget theories--I'll just get what I want."   People these days defy all authority even that which they have decided to follow. The fast will dissolve that ego, man's biggest obstruction. With ego in your way you're   missing all the benefits you said you wanted for yourself: championship, a perfect body, a keen mind, world success and great prosperity. You must build character in pursuit of these things and fasting is the fastest to afflict self. This is the way to humble the ego to automatically get to God's infinite power.

MEAT FREEZERS AND SOUL-SQUEEZERS

Many Atkins or paleo-dieters love to eat meat but hate to fast. I joined a discussion list on the internet and got tired of the constant carnal talk of meat-eating like all the meats they had stored in the freezer. When I mentioned fasting the whole group turned against me. People can eat meat but they can't fast. The hunter eats meat to survive, but then he fasts until the next (unpredictable) kill. This diet--the true diet of man--is so appetite-suppressing one can go joyfully a day or days without any thoughts of food. Fasting is a lost art and a way to great joy and quick progress. To fast is not to deprive, but to gain. The fast is the true feast but you can have both in the same day.

No one is happy eating all day long. The lack of such behavioral boundaries destroys happiness--laxness is laziness. The mind can never stay focused which is the very key to success. The formula for success is: (1) eliminate all distraction, then (2) focus.   If you're ever going to mind travel or talk to God it's going to be when you're 100% there in the spirit not the flesh with all of its appetites and cravings.   By fasting, inspiration—wisdom, knowledge and good information--flows in. By emptying the space you create an empty vacuum for something far greater to fill. This is the principle of pneumaticity: creating the "air" space which then fills in with the new. The Fast Formula is: fast to be full-filled.

BEFORE THE FOUNDATIONS OF WORLD

God planned your whole destiny before the foundations of the world. It's all there: the blueprint that goes way beyond what you could ever believe or conceive. This plan is so exciting using all your talents. This purpose and destiny for your life will bring you the greatest joy you could ever know, so don't get stuck in detours because of food obsessions. Besides the time, money and energy food makes decades go by in a blur. Get your energy up out of the gut into the brain, the enlarged brain. Fast and find this beautiful life--to be thrilled and of enormous help to humanity. Get ready to make an amazing new dent in this world. And are you ready to live the good life--the class of your highest calling? Make plans for your castle for you shall have it.

21

MINI-FASTING

Eat Once Daily—Change
with God's Speed

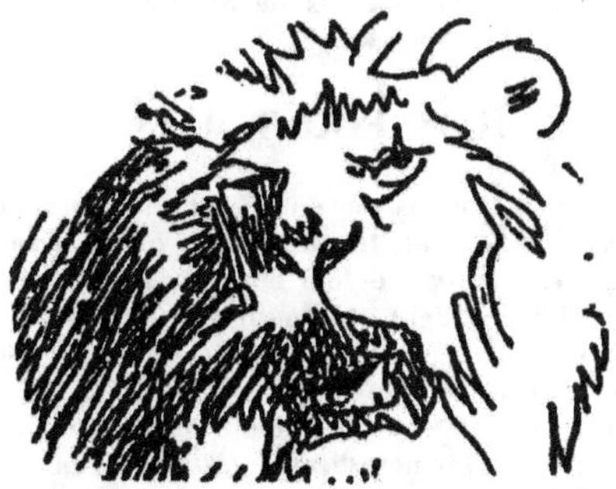

Many have so zapped their metabolisms through eating disorders that now one meal fills the bill but two starts to kill. Mini-fasting is eating once daily then fasting 24 hours. No one needs to eat more than once daily and it accomplishes so much that if done daily the health benefits are cumulative and soon you have superior health or "super-health." Superior health is the claim and promise of pure fruitarianism but I have experienced this as fallacious. It is fruit and fat like figs, nuts and cheese combined with the fast that works so well for life one doesn't need a long-term fast. The thought of a long fast is so intimidating that few ever do it or they do it once then never stop talking about it. Fasting should be just a regular routine not a "feather in your cap." With the mini-fast you can fast and receive all the many benefits but still work and play. The fast is fun. The fast works fast. The fast is union with God, the giver of all things. The mini fast is always rewarded as much as the long one.

CHAMPION GUIDES

Higher paleo daily fastarians are very happy people. For me, after so many low-vibrational years on low-fat diets this simple diet solved all riddles and gave energy and satisfaction for the day. It took so many years of suffering to return to the only way that worked in my teens when eating instinctively. I ate a huge cheese omelet each morning and was at my best and most productive as I fasted to the next day. But then theory and dogma caught hold as I listened to other people and abandoned all fat.   It took me half a life to return to the beginning when things worked best unconsciously and instinctively.

TRUE NOBILITY

If I have gut pain from fasting I'm accomplishing something knowing that area is cleaning and that self-affliction gets to God's power. Dissolve the ego by refusing to give into its wants, needs and cravings. The pain is only temporary, instantly gone when that area cleans out. Have courage, fortitude and true nobility—just skip dinner. Go for it--you'll see the great results tomorrow. There have been numerous cases of people seeing depression, fear and schizophrenia lifted completely and quickly in just one day. That's the reason to fast today--for how you'll feel tomorrow. The 24-hour mini-fast creates astounding changes. The difference in how one looks, feels, acts or conducts his talents is so vastly different while fasting that it becomes his good addiction. It's the incredible results that addict: Fasting is the old-fashioned and right way of losing weight.

JUST FOR TODAY

Just fast today and the problem is on its way out. That means zero food, not a morsel. Not eating anything will really change you to the extent that you've been a compulsive nibbler (a grape, a nut etc). Your personality and your body but particularly your soul is about to change radically. You will lose weight but you'll also lose many other non-essential or troublesome facets of your psyche. You'll be able to find things lost and do things still undone. Baby-boomers--do you feel you're getting old? Fasting is the way to level the playing field. There will be no more envy or feeble-fretful attempts to compete with youth. Whereas before you were over the hill now through fasting you can compete with anyone no matter how rich, beautiful, popular or powerful.

While Ramadan fasting is from dawn to dusk the mini-fast is from breakfast-to-breakfast, lunch-to-lunch or dinner-to-dinner. It's twenty-four hours at a time. I've always loved the breakfast plan, of getting the entire "food time" over before dawn. My days are filled with miraculous creative activity because all this energy/time waste is behind me. First you enjoy your morning with just juice or your usual morning drink. This is a very creative and busy time. Then you enjoy your fatty meal eaten slowly and luxuriously over a couple hours. Then you lavish the day immensely in a very even-keel then sleeping like a log when there is most hunger (when the height of cleansing is occurring). This is a situation where great pain is greater gain. As each mini-fast day passes you will find it much easier and will see a younger face in the mirror. This makes it easy becoming a lifetime faster with all the benefits and rewards that accrue.

FASTING FOR LIFE

As he gets older the faster doesn't have the same maladies he sees in his peers.   The wise man does today what is good for tomorrow while the fool does whatever he wants today and to hell with tomorrow. Just for today don't eat and you'll be amazed at how much easier digestion and elimination feels each new day. The effect of the highly-potent brunch will be so exhilarating and nourishing. I want to fast each day for I have discovered that eating though pleasurable pales compared to fasting, the true feast. Fruitarians who eat fruit all day yet never feel satisfied find it hard to fast as they're always in craving mode. Now on the proper diet--the one making most metabolic sense--you'll thank God for the privilege of fasting and the knowledge you have as the reason for doing it.

It's an upside-down kingdom: what is viewed as pain is actually gain. It is a privilege to fast for it's the method designed by God to get to His power. This is the anointing--the tangible presence of God which lifts all burdens and destroys all yokes. It sets the prisoners free in an amazing miracle putting you in another world, a true ascension to a much higher, more cornucopic reality. You'll see a truce to all quarrels and find--or replace with a better substitute--all that's been lost. What a wonder to watch your beauty arise and blossom.

TWO WORLDS

All the childish things we did to find favor and approval! How inefficient compared to the easy fast which works so fast seeing great healings, favor with man and achievements each day--there simply is no other way. You must anticipate the fast and be grateful as you watch your magic vistas open up. Isn't it wonderful having this trump card (when all else fails) every single day for life? There is no more need to fear, rant or rave for we have found the key-lock for a perfect life.   See the environment   radiate with new possibilities and opportunities as the world becomes your arena.   But through food addiction and preoccupation it becomes your hell or prison to be avoided--yes they are diametrically opposed these two worlds, and you can switch your whole destiny today.   Food and digestion is the basis of most of our problems.

Most psychological therapy is on the wrong page for the fast is what changes the mind and mood. The irritation of food, fat or fullness finds fallacious reasons for fear or frenzy as the frontal cortex justifies all foolish food-related acts. It makes you a phony: as it weakens, the ego must buttress up the psych through image--bragging and bull. These masks dissolve in fasting as there's no more need to build up to a false position for the new power within is as a tidal wave! No need to brag--the power is now just to be. There's no more reason to indulge in foolish flattery of supposed superiors for now the faster is on top. When you see the real power in public, the real elevation of your work and thought life fasting will become your insurance plan for life--the reality you return to with the slightest trouble or pain. In this generation that may be very often as the computer world is filled with petty and persistent problems to repair--but with fasting you won't be pulling out your hair.

Eating just once a day will be a dream come true as it makes mountains back into molehills. We all have enemies inside and out and fasting overcomes all of them. Just try it--fast at those irksome or troublesome characters and see how fast the inversion of systems occur: this is when the top becomes the bottom and the bottom the top. So I say: sail on captain for the world ahead, for you now have reason to believe all the stories you've read! Everything you want will now happen through you, a masterpiece using God's timeless method. You'll go from "no it can't be done--I'm over the hill." To "yes it can be done--I'm just beginning still."

PSYCHIC OPENING

Suddenly those sinuses open up. The whole brain explodes in a psychic opening or aperture syndrome. This is a gift of God to the unwise--the past is gone as the Tao moves on and all templates, addictions and bad memories dissolve. It was only dead habit and useless food that kept you hooked and down, so fast and move on! The bible says there are some sins that will only go out through fasting and there is no other way. You will change, transform, transfigure and the past will dissolve as a dream. You will soon see how food and habit made you delusional as it weakened and then kept you hooked to people, habits, excess and a compendious body fill with non-essential superfluity. Just fast and then say: "blubber be gone" and it will.

TIGHT THIGHS

Ladies take a look at your thighs. You see the pits that resemble the face of the moon? That's fat deposits pressing on cells filled with useless water. Both come from insulin elevation or storage mode. Eating fat without carb won't lay it on like that. It also comes from eating too much/too often. I have met many Atkins dieters who had fat thighs from eating three protein meals a day. The system must be free of food to do the miraculous things I describe. Try the 24-hour plan and see it daily diminish, for you can have tight thighs again. Just nourish the body with protein then sculpt it with leg exercise like biking or fast-walking. Watch the blubber rock n' roll, take note and watch it tighten each day. Fast, walk fast, be proud. You'll never be jealous of other (younger) women again.

IT CAN BE DONE
Beauty, Brilliance and Bounty

Fasting, I can be anything I want. To the faster the sky's the limit and there is no competition. There are no "blues" for adequate fat means fasting without hunger and weakness. Fasting evens the field--you can now compete with the younger, brighter, richer and more popular for you have God on your side and your energy in the head as opposed to the adversary who like most people is probably eating the wrong thing, too much, too often. How can you transcend? Just eat right, then don't eat.

What you're supposed to look like is: you, minus food. You're the unique blueprint which will hit the mark only when free of food. When eating the "you" is endlessly mutable, changing constantly with promiscuous eating--as does the reaction of other people to you. Every choice we make brings results and fasting always brings good ones. Just one day-fast or one meal skipped can be worth a million: from dawn to dusk (Ramadan) or the best mini 24-fast which accomplishes more. After my meal there is no thoughts of eating again as the "hunger habit" daily diminishes. You may have trouble starting the mini-fast with fruit which excites craving too much. I want to be in solid ketosis and that means fat. Now there is no excuse to eat again and you can just enjoy continuous revelations of your fasting day.

THINK BIG—THE BIGGEST

Suspend all judgment about anything until you've fat-fasted. Think only of God during the entire day: this is thinking big--the biggest. Allow your imagination of future glory and endless possibilities to run wild. Expand your boundaries. It feels so good to be released from mental restrictions and hunger-cravings. If eating the mind is always going on tangents and other procrastinations to fail. If fasting after only fruit the craving distracts to "insane" levels. Eating per se is an instant pleasure which becomes a ceiling on your thoughts: it's a fleshy up, then a down. Just think of fame and fantasy--a continuous movie script of the best you can conceive. Let your mind swing into infinity, let it go to the fat moment where past and future unite in the middle of all-time. Open your mind to transcend all the petty details of your mundane life.

You won't fear time passing any longer because the more time passes the more you've accomplished being on the fast. The more days on this routine the more blessings fall on the physical, mental and emotional. And the financial all comes clear to eventual perfection— nothing happens overnight but with each day all areas of your life improve and it's all cumulative. Your success is like a flower blossoming and much of it may be unnoticed until one day you wake up and it's a whole field: brick upon brick the building is finally complete. And not by a cheat for through the fast it is destiny you meet. If you're on the one-meal-a-day plan then you're a continual faster and that means being continuously rewarded. Then right after you eat you're right back into your fast for another day. Your virtually always fasting: You eat and then you don't eat for a long time of inspiration.

LUNCH CRUNCH—LOOSE YOUR HUNCH

That lunch though light will pull you down. You'll get to where you don't want to come down from the high fast   so you'll postpone it more on your morrows. As each day passes your digestion, assimilation and elimination is that much better. You feel better and each day's a greater accomplishment. Bloated? Say bye-bye to bloat for it's mere appearance-in-transition. Each day less total load (on the immune system) means less bloat. As you sit on and upon the bloated butt and thighs for the last time don't dismay but relate universally to all womankind of bloated thighs--you must experience it to understand what they feel, to help keep them on an even keel. Just say "Fast and daily reduce total load--soon you're on a fantastic new road".

After twenty years of fruitarianism and the protein malnourishment it brought I experienced a terrible time with food decisions. I needed protein and fat but eating meat? I was entering territory previously forbidden. My guilt added to the negative reactions. Finally I decided that the main point was just the fat and fasting which always works to bring me back to self and God. Fasting is most important so let the fat be whatever you want for that one meal--just eat and note the symptoms.   Keep trying to find the fat that works, then fast for the day so all will be made clear. Make fasting the predominant part of your life.

VEGETARIAN TRENDS

If one is reared on meat but then goes vegan that means the body adapted to sufficient protein and fat only to lose it as an adult. That's when a sharp and handsome up-and-coming-kid becomes a sagging, haggard, mid-aged loser! What happened? He started eating a so-called "balanced diet" (the usual high carb using pasta, rice, cereals) thus losing all his true balance. What a shame losing so many years to delusion, thinking mostly grains/fruits and vegetables were more "spiritual."   These cult-like made-up conceptions of what constitutes "spiritual" are very hypnotizing. What makes man truly spiritual is having the correct macronutrient ratio which then makes him truly himself--as superb as he can be. What makes man spiritual is a properly fat-fed brain which is then receptive to higher thoughts--not eating fruit all day then chanting while the brain rots.

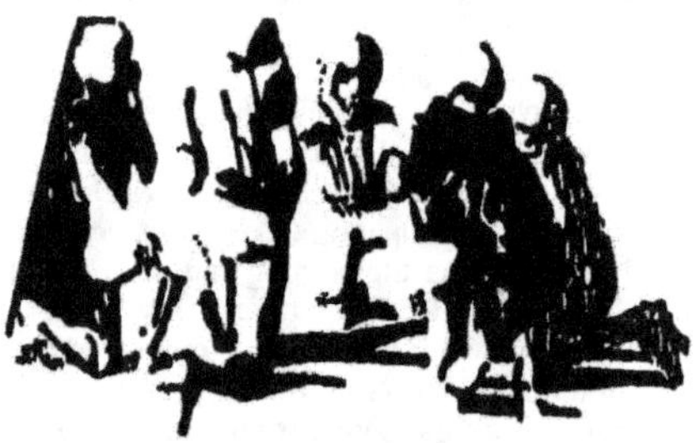

Becoming a "balanced eater" is when someone who was tough with a good immune system suddenly became susceptible and sensitive to every bug or chemical around. That's when all his friends and family say "what happened to Joe? He was so great as a kid—kind, gentle and cute." One can become that way again by reverting to the childhood diet of fauna for fat and protein are immune-enhancers. My life degraded losing protein: I went from slick and svelte to sickly and scrawny. As the world trends are going more vegan meat-eaters are often attacked by those "gentle" vegetarians. In these times bad is called good and good bad: abstainers from meat are seen as "moral" and meat-eaters "immoral." To adapt to this counterfeit philosophy (outmoded by modern science) they lose their health. I too was stuck in that brainwashing and turned against family and world which came back at me even harder being in a weakened state where I could not defend myself. Having lost connection to my world I lost my mind. Let this go and you'll feel indescribably better when finally getting what you're supposed to via fat and protein and then later the addition of fruit and when completely healed using higher paleo.   The body will be so well-nourished the fast becomes a blissfully inspired time.

EVERYONE'S A FARMER

CHAMPION GUIDES

Look around--they're all fat. It's because they're on the modern "healthy" diet filled with grains and produce mixed with some fat. Through all those starchy items they may be getting well over 200 carbs daily throwing the meat and fat into over-storage--they get fat. This is the farmer diet the AMA have agreed to advance (from outer vegan pressure): the low or no-fat high refined carb diet. Think of all that bread and jam which women take so much pride in making and baking. Then all the produce they eat makes them think it's all cleared out (it's obvious it isn't yet not to them). Now compare that to the correct ratio of 85% fat and protein and only 15% carb plus fasting each day. Perhaps now you can see how the champs will prevail, how we differ from the chimps and why the chumps have bumps.

HUNTER   GATHERER   GYPSIES

The Egyptian farmers were fat. They stayed in one place, in big families and broad communities—the butcher, the baker and the candlestick-maker. People get sick in this environment of mass production of non-paleo foods like grains.   In exact contrast is the hunter who is a slim gypsy and an artistic traveler with universal not parochial ties. He eats a meal of game and tomorrow's a meal of berries. The persecution by static society for gypsy nomads is a fact, as the difference in diet is so drastic it becomes a radical split in everything from personality to culture bringing mass persecution. If one just wants fauna "white society" may rebel in disgust. They think multi-varieties work best and hunting and gathering is unnatural. Can you imagine the hunter taking so much trouble with all those inessential side-dishes? Can you see the Paleolithic champion eating rice, beans and bread with his kill?

FASTING   RECAP

Fasting, you'll fit God like a glove. Eating you may be missing entirely. The more fine and accurate your job the more important it is to be fasting to get the gold seal of protection. If you're one of those champions who are designed to be and look best fasting, everything else will make you inferior to that state. As soon as you make the right choice God backs you up so never take counsel from eaters who don't understand or New Age folk hypnotized by the plant food route. This lifestyle is only for the very special champions who need an edge in the face of copious competition compelling them to eat right to win.

One 60-hour fast is such an adventure any miracle can happen. Get ready, for once you've fasted once you'll be addicted for life. Spend all day in paradise. Start by not eating for a 36-hour fast. It will amaze you the benefits of just one day a week. Get thin--it's those few fast days that do it. Did you binge recently? A fast will clean it all out and more before the fat cycle began. Go ahead and eat fruit but remember that fasting is better than fruit.

Dis-fattening is a coping device. As you saw in "logic of anorexia" the lonely female under group pressure feels the survival-need to jettison all excess flesh to deal with the emergencies-at-hand. Fasting has always been such a survival measure, the trump card, the last resort--the one that works. You can be so proud that you chose fasting because very few do. Dis-fattening the body is one way to find your true self. The body is filled with the past-

-so slim down, become a completely different person and start a brand new life. Use all enemies not as stumbling blocks but stepping stones to your good.

22

FAT-FASTING

**For the insulin-resistant it is "Biologic Utopia".
The Fat-Famished Brain will Make you Insane**

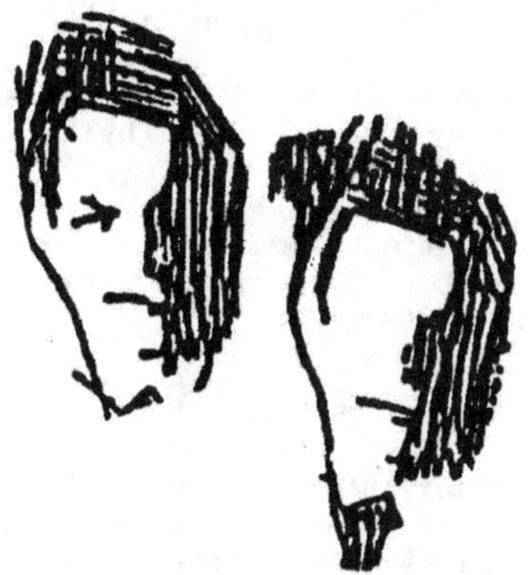

It's pure bliss living off your own fat. That's exactly what is happening when in ketosis--the state of fat-burning rather than carb-induced fat-storage. To get there just delete the fruit and expand the fats in your one meal. Now you're set-up to fly into fat-burning mode.   It has been shown that the brain and heart prefer to live on ketones for energy--not glucose— and the result is one is happier, brighter more energetic. One is always in ketosis when fasting but here's a way to make fasting a blissful no-hunger program: fat fasting. As Atkins says in regards to the treatment of extreme metabolic resistance (those who can't lose weight):

"The fasting state once induced is full of self-protective devices…like FMS [fat mobilization substance] and other lipid mobilizers leading to ketosis, loss of hunger and a variety of other benefits making the average fasting person comfortable and often exhilarated. The beautiful thing about fat is it's creating a maximal outpouring of FMS and then switching into fasting without going through the hunger/discomfort that usually characterizes the first two days". (Atkins l992*)

ENLARGED BRAIN IS COSMIC REALITY

The fantasiacal reality I wanted--like a Maxfield Parish painting of dreamy castles and beautiful landscapes--was not fruitarian as I thought, but fat-fastarian. To fly creatively high we need fat so the brain is energized-enlarged-encephalized. When combined with fasting the outcome (in consciousness) was exactly what I was seeking unsuccessfully through the fruit. Never before was I able to live on so little and finally I became the person I was supposed to be--the blueprint-design by God, eating like my ancient ancestors--"save the starch".

FRUIT IS PALEO JUST STAY FRUGAL

Did this mean all previous writings on fruitarianism need be trashed? Not at all. It seems that fruit and meat are opposites but not so if seen in the higher matrix of paleo--they go together. Especially since it has been found that man is a fat-frugivore, fruit and fat are the perfect diet or just fat with non-sweet fruit for those with IR. Reversal dieting or the marriage of Atkins and Ehret is a perfect life designed by God for man. I always have fruit with my cheese with no worries about supposed "food combining rules" we were all schooled on. Only were I to mix fat with starch would these rules apply. It is starch which kills the combo of fat and carb, not frugal fruit. I feel much more satisfied and clear after having pineapple with my cheese breakfast and they combine perfectly. One calls for the other! In food combining rules you will smother.

ISOLATION

As a fruitarian I was continuously experiencing the tyrannical constraints of interpersonal relationships--even if just intrusion on privacy--and this drove me into isolation in the desert wilderness. Though still there my whole world has opened up through higher paleo fasting. I can promise the same for you--the fruitarian trip is incredibly isolating and your whole vision will now explode into new exciting vistas. Fruitarianism or veganism is a powerful illusion that takes over the mind in a veritable hypnotic trance regarding "purity" which turns out to be disappointingly fallacious. The paleo-fatty diet will make you great so you evangelize for something new. Trying to convert the world to fruitarianism-veganism isn't a feather in your cap for you aren't doing right by inducing a failure to thrive.

Go fatarian-fastarian and people's reactions will show you you're right. Now just concentrate on listening to what God and your own instincts say--not what philosophy and ideology says. It's a very clubby atmosphere the raw foods movement--everyone smiling and looking so happy is part of the plan to convert. It isn't so great down the road--just read the bio's of ex-rawists and ex-vegans in beyondveg.com. Only the twenty-year vets can tell you the truth, not the smiling sinewy seekers you see in raw-magazines or the raw "diet gurus" raking in cash and winning admiration from their adoring foolishly fawning fans.

Listen to your instincts. Worry blocks this--worry-induced by the raw foods movement about "mucus" and cholesterol from protein-digestion which (they fail to say) the body easily deals with and eliminates while in ketosis.   Try fat-fasting. Once confirmed ignore all disconfirmers of your new direction based on physiological-metabolic truth. You may have to bid your fruitarian friends farewell for they'll only gainsay, vituperate and call you mad. You must be sure of your new position to maintain it. So many get a hold on truth only to lose it when the world crowds in with its falsely foolish philosophies. Fat is the natural diet of the human omnivore.   People are well-fitted to eat fauna, berries, leaves, vegetables and fruits. This was our diet from the beginning long before the bizarre diet habits of the 20th century plagued us. It is insulin which creates atherosclerosis as the artery wall is insulin-sensitive and promotes proliferation of arterial cells. And the lowcarb diet is completely heart-healthy--like the French who love cream, cheese and butter in just about every dish. The American view takes the opposite fat-phobic position and you must be strong to withstand the sugar-addicted mob-mentality.

RESEARCH ON FAT-FASTING

In 1961 Benoit* studied a diet that actually outdid--in eliminating body fat--the total fast by 88%. That remarkable diet provided results so spectacular that the dogmatic medicals couldn't believe their data as the diet contained 1000 calories but 90% of them as fat. The other 100 calories consisted approximately 15 grams of protein and only 10 grams of carb.

In Atkin's view nibbling works better than gorging during a fat-fast--i.e. frequent small feedings are preferable for weight loss so he divides the food allowance into four nibblings of 250 calories each. This is a fast modified for example by mouse-meals of nuts, a little cheese or guacamole—it's a method of fasting punctuated by the intake of fatty foods. I have found personally that one meal works best—I want all food behind me to maximize the blissful fasting consciousness. Fat-fasting is the most effective fat-loss diet ever described and fat is less "fattening" than protein or carb for it doesn't convert to insulin-elevating glucose and overcomes all metabolic resistance to losing weight. One is sure to go into ketosis with fat-fasting but eating carbs will suppress the production of FMS (fat mobilization substance). Let the hunter-gatherer in you come out and let starchy-sugar consumption go. You'll be so glad you found the fat-fast using mouse-meals: tiny potent bites to shrink the gut and enlarge the brain.   Doesn't this seem better then eating crates of grapes and still feeling hungry?

FAT IS NOT FINISHED

CHAMPION GUIDES

Give Your Dogs Fat Too

While the fabulous fat fast is 90% fat watch out for medical consensus panels warning us to reduce fat to 30% without exceptions! The scientists seeing the benefit of fat are banned from consensus panels who see fat--any fat (even essential fatty acids and olive oil) must never go beyond 30% of total intake. It's a sad day in medical history as many doctors are actually caving into the pressure from raw food circles and their corny magazines. We were far more advanced at the turn of the century when people ate multiple courses of fatty (delicious) meat without thought. Yet there were no heart problems until sugar, coca-cola and refined flour were unleashed on the public in the twenties. Fat-phobia overrides these facts and continues to hypnotize the public into a frenzy as it eliminates fat--yet gets fatter. Most people even eliminate fat from the diet of their poor dogs--yet another class of victims of the fat fallacy--who get fat and have a lackluster coat. My five grown dogs are as peppy as slim puppies with fur-coats as shiny as glass. Give your dog cheese and watch him beam with gratitude and love for you have finally done the right thing by this gentle loving omnivore.

FAT: TASTE AND LOOKS

What a shame for those controlled by medical society, for low-fat diets are hardly satisfying. If someone eats like a king (this means delicious fat) he doesn't have the dry skin and austere look of many vegetarians. Protein and fat gives structure to the cells and the face as it soothes, moisturizes and brings water to the surface to give that "beau-glow". Fat is predominant in world cuisine because of its luxurious satisfying taste, its richness and its capacity to satiate appetite. Fat is the food of feasts as butter, cheese and cream is the backbone of delicious fine cuisine. Like the French diet it's the yummy fat which makes everything taste so great and appetite suppression and satisfaction is its greatest virtue. My natural craving for fats was completely fulfilled through cheese in the morning as I became trim and never craved any kind of food again.   "Higher paleo" is distinguished from fruitarianism by it's view of the essentiality of FATS.

NASOLABIAL FOLDS : LOW-FAT UGLINESS

The features of low-fat dieters show dry skin, pasty complexion and deep furrows—these are the nasolabial folds from the side of the nose to the side of the mouth and below. This aged look is characteristic of low-fat intake and is hardly the look of God's image in which we are created. Tiny bites of HQ are enough to recreate daily your structure or the blueprint of what you're supposed to look like: the constellation of the energy at birth, your seed symbol. Man evolutionarily a hunter requires animal protein and this gives him his good Godly "looks". Look at the movie stars decades back--their visage and hair had real luster. This is the look of the fat and protein-satisfied man. The difference between small and huge HQ fatty meals is evidenced in the drastic transfiguration of your looks for the closer you can get to emptiness (lack of obstruction) the closer you are to the Creator's design.

FRUIT-FAT FASTING AND RED SALAD

Fruit-fat fasting is for those who wish to maintain the fruitarian way but still keep insulin low without using any animal foods. Here the benefits of this fat-fasting plan is customized to fit the fruitarian: the lowcarb red salad with avocado was the key for me. By eating this dynamite breakfast then to return to the fast for a day gave me the highest health and creativity as a pure fruitarian. You'll be eating one big, luxurious, slow meal which you can enjoy for two hours. The fresh food is most delicious and each day you'll enjoy it more as your digestive-assimilative apparatus works better. Dice two tomatoes, three red bells and avocados dressed with the juice of one lemon and olive oil with garlic powder. Though avocado is only 2.1 percent protein (as opposed to 25% for cheese) it will elicit glucagons which turns you into a fat-burning machine. It was only sugar that elevated insulin and your storage of fat. After eating this delicious non-sweet salad you'll be in highest heaven as you digest it all day.

Fruitarians over-indulging in sweet fruit may find some of the same symptoms I did over twenty years. I found out they were all from hyper-insulinism: obsession with food, habit of night eating, tendency to binge, craving for sweets and starch, compulsive eating, no food fulfillment, irritability, drops in strength, fatigue, mood swings, lack of concentration, anxiety mixed with sadness and depression, dizziness, brain fog, gastritis and bloating. After twenty years of this, these symptoms hit me every time I ate as little as an apple. It was as discouraging as it was progressive. For someone who overindulged in sweets and starch early in life the insulin receptors were so worn out that just one touch of glucose sent insulin pouring forth, dropping blood-sugar levels low (fatigue) while storing fat and water. Sludgy, stodgy, sullen and swollen I became tired, irritable, angry and hungry.

I COULD FEEL IT HAPPENING...

As a vasoconstrictor, insulin constricts all the airways and vessels. As it holds water this means hypertension as everything closes down and in. Many fruitarians have described to me this feeling of constriction as if they were having a heart attack as the "chest closed in." Look at the difference between the two states: insulin suppresses the immune system, increases inflammation and pain, decreases oxygen flow, decreases endurance and causes platelet aggregation (constricting blood vessels).   The result is breathlessness, headache, cramps, swelling and rashes. It is not fat which brings on heart attacks but carbs--in the absence of carb fat is totally harmless. Glucagons on the other hand brings a vaso-dilation (opening-up) while enhancing immunity, decreasing pain and inflammation, increasing oxygen flow and endurance, preventing platelet aggregation, dilating airways and decreasing cell-proliferation (cancer).   Cancer, heart disease, diabetes and artherosclerosis is sugar/starch based with no relation to dietary fat.

FRUIT-FAT FOR FRUITARIANS

I was still fruitarian when I decided to take this information and adapt the diet to my own metabolic needs. I deleted all sweet fruit like dates, grapes and oranges and stuck to cucumber lemon/lime tomatoes bell pepper and avocado. When you eat fat like avocado (in the absence of sugar) the body goes into ketosis marked my loss of appetite for the day, along with the release of lipid mobilizers. You're not hungry, you have an abundance of energy and burn fat which the body loves to live on. So why not take one high fruit-fat meal then go right into a miraculous day--once the red salad is digested the body automatically readapts to grasping all needed nutrition from the air and sun. Fruit fat is so wonderful as it oils the tissue system and organs, brings warmth and comfort to the body and structure to the way it fits together. It makes things right as it soothes, protects, comforts and brings radiant energy with a sheen ("divine luster") to the appearance.

FAT PHOBIA IS A CULTURAL HYPNOTIC

The prevalent panic over dietary fat is a cultural hypnotic. It makes no sense scientifically once one knows the metabolic processes that follow the eating of fat vs. carb. We should be a lot more afraid of being fat but not at all afraid of dietary fat when eating low carbs—or even when eating sweet fruit if followed by the fast. Someone may start on this high-fat/low-carb fruit diet and be enormously happy with it only to be talked out of it by friends. The fat-phobia against even avocado and olive oil is the biggest example of social hypnotism I can think of. If one eliminates all fat from the diet the only things left are vegetables, starch and sugars—how sad! Many vegetarians are fat, for the consequences of eliminating fat and then gorging on starch and sweet fruit along with salads are devastating. Never have we had such an obese nation of adults and children. Fortunately non-sweet fruit is very delicious—tomatoes, squash, peppers, cucumbers, avocado and olive are so freshly tantalizing. I see this marriage of Atkins and Ehret (fat and fruit) as a most fitting and wonderful solution for a happy long lustrous life.   And since the colon demands fats to work properly the daily evacuation makes life a continuous vacation.

HOW THE FRUITARIAN MOVEMENT HURTS

The fruitarian movement has bought into the same old fallacy of fat phobia (putting down avocados and olive oil) and complete naiveté about sugar. Since most fruit is sweet they fear to investigate the bad effects of insulin from fructose and gainsay anyone who brings up the point. So they say to avoid fats--"it's not fruitarian to eat fats" or "all fats are acid-forming"--thus conforming to the current politico-medically correct line of thought that fat is the culprit to all things. But the fruit fat olive doesn't create acid--it's the fastest eliminator of it--so what exactly is their basis other than how things "seem" devoid of true science reasoning? They, like the culture at large have a knee-jerk reaction to the mere word "fat" without any understanding of the metabolic processes which follow the ingestion of fat vs. sugar and starch.

The fruitarian movement would do well to accept and absorb fats into the diet they are propounding. To not do so is to encourage a failure to thrive in millions of people across the world.

23

FAUNA-FASTING

**No Fruit Just Fauna. Many have so ruined their
metabolisms from incorrect diet they become
pure fatarians with little or no carbohydrate.**

Man is a fat-frugivore. He is first a fat-eater with the ability to eat fruit. But the faunivore human is one whose ability to eat fruit was damaged. If through a history of overindulgence in fruit, starch and sugar he developed hyperinsulinism the case may be he ends up a pure faunivore, an exclusive eater of animal foods and herbs.   So although all men are fat-frugivores the ratios of fat to fruit may change. Some people are more like the apes: frugi-faunivores i.e. mainly fruit-eaters with biological adaptations to eat fat.   The faunivore human has found that animal protein and fat are essential to his health but carbs aren't. the following is Peter's self-discovery after embarking on one cheese omelet meal a day or every two-three days:

Hi Karen. I love Paleo-Fasting. It has changed my life and made me so happy every day.   It gives me so much energy and enthusiasm. I was a dull log but now I'm so excited I can't sit quiet.   I don't want to go back to my former diet and I've ceased discussing this with anyone for they would only deny it.   I just feel too good now like I'm going places. Now I'm able to fast 60 hours after an omelet and it s wonderful.   I wake up in the morning with so much energy ready to take down the world feeling between paradise and eternity.   Thanks to you for showing me how to fast. Ciao your friend for life Pietro

The fasting combined with fat results in tiny tummy and brainy brilliance. After one year of fat-fasting into complete metabolic recovery I can enjoy the fat-frugivorous diet--the reversals between detox (grapecure) and rebuilding (fat) is a wonderful lift and a divine gift.

But first I had to counterbalance the sugar-inundated system with exclusive fauna fasting for one year.

TINY TUMMY BRAINY BRILLIANCE

Hyper-sensitives can really feel how carb stimulates fat storage and other profound metabolic hormonal changes. Hyperinsulinism which crams fat into cells and water logs the legs into "tree trunks" is so hereditary that one must go the other way to achieve balance: Delete the carb-component and one's life and looks change dramatically for the better. As it is genetic he suddenly doesn't resemble anyone in his whole family—amongst white pasty polar bears there is one shiny sorrel steeple!

Seem strange? Remember that all great truths began as blasphemies.   Protein and fat is fully and nutritionally complete for the human omnivore but over the last 30 years we've been severely brainwashed to eat predominantly produce with grains resulting in obesity and the other degenerative diseases of civilization (see "forbidden seed"). We're on the wrong page and its getting worse as the government and medical "consensus panels" chime in under pressure from raw-foodists campaigns over the internet.   The hunter vs. farmer skeletons tell all.

MEAN (FAT-FAMISHED) RAWFOODISTS
Don't Get Drawn In!

Don't get drawn into the raw food movement. Every time I got involved with rawfoodists I witnessed anger, rage and rudeness. It's really quite unbelievable since one would "think" they would be the gentlest on earth if what they say about meat-eating is correct and true-- namely that it creates violence and just eating raw food makes one gentle. Not true. The fat-deprived brain becomes uncontrollably violent especially when combined with sugar- inundation and bloat from eating so much high-water sweet fruit. Also they are depriving themselves of categories of food they want or need. Diet dogma is destructive. Eat raw when you can, but of primary importance is your fat and protein needs. Paul Bragg taught us this—he weekly ate a piece of fish though he ate raw produce most of the time. Fat connects you to spirit and properly fuels thy brain, heart, glands and certainly skin. You'll see a sheen and become quite lean. You'll feel keen—but all-raw and no-fat means mean. The hostile encounters I've had with rawfoods groups have been despicable and unrepeatable. What they have I do not want.

I myself found that produce confused things as I was recovering from such drastic fat and protein deprivation. Dry skin became smooth and moist during the fat-fast but became dry again when going the other way. Damaged metabolisms usually evince malabsorption syndrome—the food goes out as it went in.   That means raw vegetables become excruciatingly uncomfortable to digest—I'll never forget waiting all day to feel good again, praying it would just move down. But fat was so smooth it nourished and revived the system. What a paradox! When I regained metabolic balance only fruit worked with fat—not thorny vegetables--and I became a very happy fat-frugivore, the way man was designed to eat. For the true faunivore human   plants are much harder to digest than meat so there they sit and the whole process bogs down. It may seem incredible after all the brainwashing about the necessity of eating mostly plant foods. But the transformation of some into perfect health by fat is so powerful they never want to "change categories" from fat to carb again—the effect is so evident they never want to be "kicked out of ketosis".

SMALL MEALS PUNCTUATING THE FAST

In the one type of paleo-fasting you're actually fasting all the time punctuated with bites of fruit or fat. While recovering, plant food will be impossible to digest and as Billings says meat is so much easier in prehistory it was always eaten separately. So much for natural "hygienic" instructions to always eat them together! Atkins found that the least likely thing people are allergic to is meat. I once knew a hypersensitive who after years of promiscuous eating and bulimia zapped the immune system so much that she became a universal reactor to all food--she learned her "ugliness" was just reaction. When she started to eat fruit, nuts or dairy followed by fasting her reactions lessened daily. She learned how the effect of today's food is solely determined by her total load on the immune system yesterday. All the fat and protein she was eating enhanced immunity. Fat-satisfied at last, on the fast she ceased thinking of food and her reactions and started attending to angels, animals and ancestral logic. Her health improved overnight and she became fascinated with the infinite world beyond eating. This incredible release from addiction is the auto-reaction to eating the correct diet from the beginning for man.

WITHDRAWAL FROM COMFORT FOODS

When you don't get your allergic comfort food (carbs) you'll get fatigued (withdrawal) and think you need it or have to have it: At first you may feel sleepy and fatigued as the system isn't used to low carb/high fat, but in under a week you'll be swinging, having gone through the fire as the new enzymes are established and the old comes out allowing room for the new. A whole new bloodstream and normal balance will create real pep--the heightened energy of the Neolithic hunter. Sleep on and look forward, for the fat-fast is completely pain-free. You may even ask "are things really happening?" Yes, but you don't realize it because there is no hunger.

CLEANSING REACTIONS

Fat can be frightening due to the generational fears surrounding us. I gave up telling people what I was doing as I experienced weird cleansing reactions from predictably in this order: the intestine, the lungs then the skin. When fat-fasting (one small morning meal) these amazing events occurred: (1) intestines: I took colon cleansing herbs--psyllium husk, ginger and alfalfa leaf powders and eliminated 50 feet of mucoid plaque--""ropes"--in one week. The abdomen suddenly became very flat. (2) lungs. Then I had asthma and productive coughing for a week after which that area cleared as glucagons dilated all airways. My breathing became deep and clear. (3) skin. A "week of welts" all over the body followed as the skin system elimination took over from the completed intestinal-lung cleansing. Every cell "dumped" years of carb build-up and I resembled someone with measles--the way a high-energy engine (like a child) eliminates quickly.

I felt and looked so different after this magnificent and magical reconfiguration, and knew it was the beginning of a new life as old layers unpeeled back to the root. My entire scalp itched intensely and the hair became suddenly fuller and the shape of the head longer and narrower. After this three-week rite of passage I realized I had rebuilt and cleansed the body while eating only fauna-animal foods and fasting. As soon as this started happening I decided to facilitate the process by reducing the one meal to a tiny bit of fat. The process quickened and all cells unscrambled, dumped and reconfigured. The reward was a whole new body built with HQ—the highest quality food. Bloating may occur as the cells dump and the body holds water to dilute the poison—just endure as you're almost there, as you go from mesomorph (a bit rounded) to ectomorph (sharply defined thin and flat). You have reached that point in the cleansing and rebuilding process where the morphology--size and shape--has completely changed.

FUN FABULOUS PAIN-FREE FAT-FASTING

It's so inefficient to be hungry all the time or have to eat again—so eat fat to not be hungry while you burn fat. I want only to fast each day to be close to God and see all the miracles happening: they're always there but with all our energy down in the gut who can apprehend them all?   But staying high it's one magic coincidence after another. When I began introducing this concept in groups everyone wanted to argue against it—they want to eat two or three meals a day out of pure fear of what feels like "nothingness" to them. The truth is they're using food as entertainment--a device to avoid anxiety. But this fear will soon be replaced with miraculous insights and excellent work habits. You will learn to love the fast more than the feast which only brings energy down from the higher world.

3 SYSTEMS: DIGESTIVE OR ELIMINATIVE ENERGY?

Once we're into the fast we shouldn't eat one thing for there are three systems: digestive, assimilative and eliminative. 85% of our energy is in one or the other and it can't be in more than one. If you let the sequence go through you'll have amazing elimination the next day as the energy stays high in the head. If one is fasting the 85% of available energy for digestion automatically now shifts to assimilation (clear beautiful skin) and elimination (each morning a huge package). This was so anti-dogma it was a veritable science discovery. Even while eating "binding" cheese for the one meal the evacuation was made perfect from the daily fast. The truth is the colon needs fat and with energy vested in elimination the results are a miraculous "cleansing". If we're into the eliminative phase--only to eat again--the system must go back to digestion, but if we allow the sequence to go through we are eliminating all the debris that makes one ugly—"ordinary".   With the breakfast-only (Ramadan) plan I became skinny--not scrawny, but more like a gazelle: quick and taut, shiny and fawnlike because it was all-elimination all day long.

The fruitarian became a fawn only after electing this temporary life of fat-fasting. Until then evacuation was unstable and the body showed protuberances.   Forget all the constant food issues and arguments, just stay with one fatty meal and go right into ketosis and fasting. You'll see it's fun to fast in a much higher state of perception and problem-free existence. All is overcome and all is made clear as the total load (on the immune system) is daily reduced and each day you are bloating less. You're entering a whole new life separate from the mass. You'll see the astounding implications of the heavy-carb diet--of that other world where just about everyone is fat. You'll begin to notice all the hodgepodge people place in their shopping carts, how fat has become the norm and how you are advancing towards a sleek futuristic appearance—no more forlorned.

FASTING AND TIMES OF DAY

I love the seasons of the day. In predawn mornings I love the one meal followed by energetic but calm creative work.   At noon I'm "off" and listen to music or some other means of relaxation and inspiration in the "aft-fast".   Only in leisure--when "off"--can I really appreciate these things. There is a total difference depending on the mode we are in how the senses effect us. It is the times of day and your peak periods vs. leisure that will determine when you eat your one meal and when you do your most creative work--when it's effortless. Paradoxically it is always when I'm "off" that instantly the creative is unleashed. Yes only in leisure does it blossom. Leisure makes the creative artist busy all day so optimize each moment to the spirit of fasting after your one meal. I don't want "frequent nibbling" as Atkins advised for then I'm missing the highest thoughts from the skies! The "aft-fast" is a blast.   "Fat" means spirit and this tremendous power and glory is infused as heaven aligns with earth through fasting--your emptiness attracts higher vibration. Then energy stays in the head while the world is stuck in the gut and need to "suck up". That fat becomes an electrical conduit to the source.

STAYING SLIM WHILE FILLED TO THE BRIM

Staying slim is a worldwide goal and it's a constant problem keeping fat off the frame. The anorexic has already felt so battered by the world of big people she must stay slim for whatever self-image she has left.   This is a perfect plan to stay slim and fun-fast without dire results. Some people have not been successful getting slim on three meals a day as the legs become tree trunks indicating too much toxicity. In this diet I am advancing mini-fasting is critical—after an initial cleansing crisis you'll be slim for life with no toxic reactions. It's the localization of all eating into one meal that does the trick. I was a skinny (scrawny) fruitarian but when turning to the Atkins diet was dismayed at the rolls of fat on chest, backside, thighs. Only the fast worked and adding fruit after recovery sealed the deal in a tremendous way to feel.

FAST FOR ELIMINATION INTO SUCCESS

The formula is: all disease is obstruction, all recovery elimination bringing all success by attraction. You're coming up to the finish line. For perfect success on Monday I'm prescribing a two-day 60-hour fast from Friday to Monday morning's predawn meal. You can be so blue, jealous, angry, bloated, constipated or wrecked (recovering from a binge) on

Friday. But then you embark on your two-day fat fast and you've now stepped into a new world. It's this realization alone which releases PHF so as early as Saturday your reality changes to joy by intention alone. Then just look forward to champion status Monday a.m. Be happy—you must fast first and now you're doing it. Right from the outset you experience the black and white difference between your inferior (lower fleshly) and fasting (higher spiritual) self—not on Monday but as soon as Saturday by your intention alone.   What a joyous life: daily fruit-fat-fastarianism.

If you've been carb-binging (carbs being the "normal" binging food according to Parade) then you likely need a sledge-hammer to get through the cemented intestine. Sugar and starch hits the gut like lead for when one binges like that just the combo of bread and jam will create cement. You'll find that eating normally won't break through--only fasting with herbs (like psyllium and bentonite) breaks the block--it's that serious. At this transition time the sludge contents of sugar and starch actually does you a favor acting as an appetite-suppressant like having a pillow in the stomach! But thank God that with each moment the bulldozer is moving the mountain. Congratulations. You've now embarked on the real vacation of your life, one with guaranteed rewards.

DELETE THE THRIFTY GENE

I have met modern Egyptians who were fat, having inherited the thrifty gene from the days of the Pharaohs when they were plagued with famines. I too inherited a thrifty gene and yet have little fat, having made the gene inoperative through the elimination of starchy carbs and too much food. If hyperinsulinism and the thrifty gene is hereditary your whole family may be very fat while one member is brown and ultra-thin with low-carb high-fat and fasting—thus pulling the plug on the thrifty gene. Deleting carb makes it null, void and of none effect! The no-hunger fat-fast is much more fun than the feast for fasting is letting go of earth and soaring to the heights where all things are now possible. Fat-fasting is no-hunger energy and bliss.   If you want a piece of fruit half way through the day's fast try it and note the symptoms. If its ok enjoy your fat-frugivorous life of bliss. But as I was healing and regaining lost balance the hunger it evoked was not worth it. I wanted to stay even in a state of non-craving having nothing to do with will-power. After a year of this kind of ketotic sailing I finally achieved the True Diet of Man,   the Biblical diet of the Holy Land: raisins, figs, nuts, cheese—and leaves and fish on occasion.

A Ramadan fast would be just skipping lunch each day--fasting 7 meals a week. Have a breakfast of fat and fruit if you want and if still hungry nuts or cheese. You won't be hungry until night. This makes fasting so easy you won't even consider yourself fasting but will just enjoy your day maximally productive until dinnertime. Fasting is so beneficial: you'll witness miraculous debt-cancellations, finding things lost, solving all problems and attracting what you want—miracles. That's fasting and you get there through fat and the Neolithic diet to which we are perfectly adapted.

FAT FOR IMMUNITY AND MAXIMUM DIGESTION

Since fat is easier than plants to digest, cultures eating mostly meat with only 5% carb show no heart problems, diabetes or obesity. Undigested food pockets and a body filled with debris is so immuno-suppressed disease takes over. The fauna-faster is fasting on fauna, cheese or eggs as one would fast on grapes. What looks like counter-cleansing when viewed through the detox matrix is actually a way of staying in ketosis where the fun is, since you're living on your own fat which is the highest energy (ketones). The brain and heart loves this fat and you'll see the skin and glands like it too as all rashes, dryness and wrinkles from incomplete assimilation and elimination are replaced by soft moist youthful skin, vigor and superior immunity.

The more fat (in relation to carb) you eat in the one meal the higher the "ketotic ratio" and the more appetite-suppressive, energetic and easy the fast will be. You are now living on the fastest diet known to man as the fat-fast works 80% faster than a water fast. The body tends to collect fat especially with the thrifty gene but a no-carb fat deletes that problem: Since fat-with-carb is the biggest elevator of insulin,   delimiting plant food works very well for as the ketotic ratio of fat to carb lowers, the magic is lost. Keeping the ketotic ratio high (without produce) means the fat melts right into the body and the "tight" satisfaction takes over for the day--the hunger trap is sealed and replaced with energetic satisfaction.

HAPPY FATARIANS

What a paradox that after twenty years seeking purity through fruit I would end up recovering by eating animal fat. It was a contradiction being so restricted as a fruitarian (the "superior diet") yet remaining scrawny and wasted--but now I had remarkable health as the body achieved structure and glow. Yet it meant constant collision with culture since most of the public and physicians agree with either the high-carb low fat diet including grains or the lowcarb diet—but not a life of constant reversals between both.   Temporarily only the fauna of one cheese omelet a day took the collapsed shack to a sturdy castle and once deficiency burnout ended I again craved fruit. This is neat, predictable and logical.

INSUBSTANTIAL MANNA VS. EARLY AMERICA

The wandering Izraelites wanted meat so God rained down quail--they didn't want the "insubstantial manna" of plant food. This reminds me of America early in this century. People were ashamed not bringing meat to a pot-luck as plant food was regarded as inferior. So much today are just cheap concoctions of plant food and grains. It doesn't seem insubstantial because it fills and makes fat but it falls so short of man's needs he keeps eating junk to feel satisfied. This increased craving is instigated by constantly elevated insulin and then hypertension- seeking-a-fix. The paleo potluck would be: someone brings a roast, another the leaves and dressing, another a bowl of grapes, another guacamole, another some steamed vegetables, another a desert of nuts and raisins. How much neater and efficient it is to eat whole foods—not concoctions created in kitchens--and then fast without thought or pang. Have your daily feast and then fast--an even bigger feast of inspiration and joy is coming your way today.

THE MENTAL

The new life of fasting after fat and fruit will avoid all protein/calcium deprivation as we become radically healthy creatures. The difference is felt supremely on the mental level as the brain is rightly nourished with protein and fat. True genius is a youthful mind: this is a mature mind meaning perpetually open. The immature mind is fixed, rigid, closed--it shuts down at a certain point and tenaciously clings to limited ideas. The old mind which is closed, stagnant and lifeless can happen in the teenage years while the young mind remains young by continuous nourishment from new ideas--its not afraid of new concepts or surrendering old ones.

This new and youthful mind must be complete in its unique self-expression but this enormous freedom can only be gained by fueling the engine aright. If not, the mind gets old acting in line with deception and lifeless ideas that seem so "living" and "loving" coming from "live foods" while avoiding "dead or cooked" ones. The opposite is the truth for the dead immature malnourished mind sticks to deception hypnotized by the majority view. He will go through the motions but not be truly alive--acting without imagination, originality or creativity though he may be "trendy." The dense fogged mind always falls in with the majority view or what "they" see as truth. This will no longer be true of you—the majority of the "few".

Yoga means integration and this comes from contacting and uniting with the source through the properly nourished brain. Then uniqueness shines through with true self-expression, forever becoming and eternally new. With spontaneous creativity as a vessel of God (the only source) one is always ahead because he's always himself—pure which is truly secure. Don't hold on to counterfeit dogma—let outmoded concepts like "fruitarianism" go. Fast for revelation after rightly fueling the new receptive brain. Now you are truly spiritual, being led by spirit not flesh. Being led is "prompted" as the right words arise in consciousness.

VIVA LAS VEGAS

Do you feel like life is passing you by? Do you fantasize about being in the flashy lights of Las Vegas or other sparkling places on earth? Are you dissatisfied with your present situation? I can promise you that if eating the wrong food you feel lousy no matter where you are. But with proper nourishment and fasting every minute becomes a flashing scintillating miracle as you ascend to heavenly perceptions. This is better than Vegas.

The bad eater is always on the go rushing about and traveling, searching for happier greener pastures. Dissatisfied, he never stops. The faster on the other hand needs only to stay wherever he is and just enjoy. It's called mind traveling through space where past and future unite. This mental transport far exceeds elusive gains from physical relocation or jet-setting, and what a trip! Soar to the heights after fat or fruit and then just fast while staying home like Rome: Expand the moment which becomes "fat" with new insights. Vegas is an empty though loud distraction compared to your life, your environment, your experience of the times of day and seasons. Only in your own situation is there real life as your little cabin becomes a castle.

The trick is not to "be young" but to look young when old. Anyone can look young when young so where's the achievement there? Instead, eat fat then fast to separate from crazy corn-fed cronies (be rare). Then in culture infuse your bold truth—be a scare!

KK Fat-Fasting Revelations: (1) Pain? It's got to hurt to work. (2) Fast, and take it on faith that <u>nothing happening</u> indicates everything's <u>going</u> to happen: op-truth. (3) If you're too dependent on people, it seems God will remove them. Don't attach or hang on to people—just God and He'll change the reactions of the clod.

24

FORBIDDEN SEED

High-Carb Diet killed the Egyptians

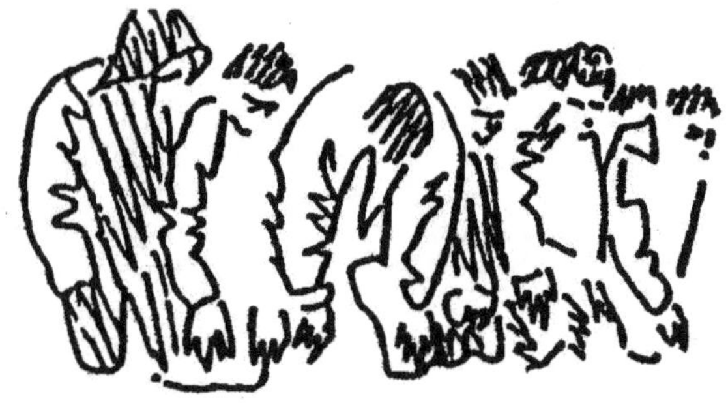

If your doctor tells you a diet of low-fat high-carb is best, watch out! Egyptians dined the same way and   died of coronary heart disease, cancer, high blood pressure, diabetes, atherosclerosis and obesity.

During the 3000 years of 2500 B.C. to 395 A.D. the Egyptians refined the art of mummification. Scientists have analyzed these mummies in great detail to determine blood type, body size and shape, bacterial or parasitic infections and diseases that caused death. Along with the extensive history of life on the Nile we know the diet of average Egyptians consisted primarily of carbs. Wheat and barley were the staple crops made into a course bread consumed in great quantities--the army was rationed five pounds of bread per day and were called the "bread eaters."

Egyptian farmers cultivated many fruits and sweetened their food with honey. They dined on bread, cereals, fruit and vegetables, some fish and poultry, almost no red meat, olive oil instead of lard and goat's milk for drinking and cheese. This is the same as our modern high-carb low-fat diet most physicians call "healthy". Though they used no refined sugar the Egyptians had terrible dental problems as teeth wore down until both enamel and dentin exposed the soft pulp. Free of enamel, the living tissue and empty canal was chronically infected and abscessed. They also showed severe gum disease despite eating no sugar--because starch in grains turns to sugar. So many vegetarians who agree sugar is bad are in denial about their precious grains.

It all seems so "spiritual": the beautiful fruits, vegetables and grains but elevated insulin is a non-spiritual state: mood-swings, fatigue, depression, irritability and constipation. The last time I indulged my bread-craving I will never forget the feeling of puffing up into fat storage. It was very difficult to breathe and I sat upon pillows for thighs. This nightmare of messed-up metabolism dissolves when switching back to fat—instantly revived, it's like coming home again. These relapses are good as they are opportunities to see the radical difference in someone with insulin resistance (IR). How many masses of miserable men in institutions and jails are really just psycho-split from the starchy diet while having IR? There are only three macronutrients: fat, protein and carb. Fat and protein go together and carb stands alone. It's the difference between a fly swatter and an atom bomb so don't ever trivialize carb or the demon of carb-craving.

DRY PALENESS VS. MOIST DARK COMPLEXION

Sugar and especially starch is the biggest lure in Americans. It never satiates or soothes as it claims--but still it beckons. Know what insulin does, take note each time you give in and soon you won't be going back. As the system stores you'll see white dust clogging all pores! Everything is swollen, dusty, pasty, round, puffy. The whole western world is bloated resembling white polar bears. Just change categories--from starchy seed products to fat and the skin becomes tightly-woven again, the basis of "dark complexion". Much "paleness" is just starchy dust from grains combined with sweet fruits (jam).

As a frugivore I felt sugar-inundated as manifested in skin dryness—this was carb-storage (called glycogen) in the skin. Another result was bloated abdomen. When I see these signs including constriction I instantly stop the fruit and reverse (escape) into fat-fasting and within hours the skin becomes moist and smooth again, the gut flat. In a few days I include fruit and all goes well once more. Knowing when to delete sugar is all part of the plan of reversal dieting, but rarely do I cut out the fat.

LOW-FAT MAKES YOU FAT

Like most Americans the Egyptians ate what the diet "experts" recommend for weight loss: fruits and vegetables and coarse whole-grain bread yet they were still very obese--not just a little overweight but super-fat! Paleopathologists describe huge folds of excess skin indicating extreme obesity in the ancient Egyptians. It certainly wasn't their beauty ideal for they painted and carved idealized pictures of slender sophisticates everywhere, just like our magazines it was just compensation or envy of something few had—elegant svelte.

We would not expect heart disease in view of their low-fat diet but again there was an epidemic of heart and vascular disease throughout ancient Egypt. The arteries of the Egyptian mummies were not smooth and supple but rather choked with greasy cholesterol-laden arteries that were calcified and atherosclerotic. The arteries were scarred and thickened indicating high blood pressure. From their low-fat diet the Egyptians were dropping dead from heart attacks! So the Egyptians were disabled by dental problems, fat bellies and deadening heart disease while cholesterol plaque and high blood pressure narrowed their young arteries into short life. And all this from whole grains and produce and a little fish and fowl. Yet we moderns are told to eat loads of whole grains, fresh fruits and vegetables to prevent or reverse these diseases.

GRAINAGE MEANS DAMAGE

Throughout history whenever man turns away from his traditional paleodiet to grain-vegetables-fruit his health has declined. Game-hunting sustained our ancestors 2 million years ago as man lived mainly on meat and fat--from 60 to 90% of his calories were from game animals, birds, eggs, reptiles and insects with only 5-10% coming from carbs. Our physiology functions optimally on fat supplemented with roots, shoots, berries, vegetables and fruits. Only within the last 100 centuries have we become mainly carb eaters only supplemented with meat: from 75 to 25% meat occurring in 400 generations--far short of the 1000 to 10000 generations needed for true genetic changes.

The change to agriculture created health problems but in pre-agricultural times--according to fossil remains--human health was excellent. People were tall and lean with well-developed, strong dense bones and sound teeth.   Tooth decay was minimal and there is little evidence of disease (Cassidy). But post-agricultural man--though his diet was more abundant and predictable--was shorter.   He had brittle bones, extensive tooth decay, mal-nutrition and chronic disease.   This general decline was felt throughout the world--from the east Mediterranean to Peru the agricultural diet brought disease and death-seen as "progress".

ELEGANT BONES MEANS "HUNTER"

Archeologists see these changes as so predictable they classify people as hunters or farmers by the state of their bones and teeth: If teeth and bones were excellent and strong they were hunters. If decayed, weak and deformed they were farmers--eating corn, beans, rice and squash with wild plants and animals only as supplements. The life expectancy of the farmers was low and infant morality very high. Children had thirteen times more infections in long bones than hunters while iron-deficiency anemia was non-existent in hunters. Think of our modern society: the degenerative diseases are rising at the same rate, all from starch they refuse to hate and fear of animal on the plate.

ANIMAL-ON-THE-PLATE

These are alarming findings as most of the world is going vegetarian high in grains, produce and fruit sugar--the Egyptian diet. When people switch from meat to a vegetarian life their "gestalt" changes from a "delicious meal" to an "animal on the plate." I can't eat meat either from this ingrained hypnotic—so much so that the mere sight or smell of meat repels. I can only eat cheese which would   not entail cruelty in a natural setting of small-farm symbiosis. But sympathy for animals which I surely have must take second place to our own good health. Protein deficiency and the signs thereof are appearing everywhere and is simultaneous with mass obesity. Its all happening as the farmer's diet replaces the healthy hunter-gatherer diet—as the mass public is obediently though blindly listening to the medical profession's warnings to eat high-refined carb with mostly produce and low or no fat. The latest consensual medical panel even says we should drop all fat even the sacred olive oil!

I can really appreciate the great harm of this since my skin looked like an old shriveled up chicken when on all-produce but became moist and youthified practically overnight when eating fat. These obvious signs indicate like changes occurring on all levels including the brain. When I finally ate fat I became normal and the persecutory phobias of fruitarianism left. The vegetarian movement has debased our bodies all due to a philosophy. Repeat many times: " I will not sacrifice my good health on the altar of ideology again."

BAKERY CRAVINGS vs. FIG-FASTING

Many wives think they're helping their husbands by making bread as replacement for fat and meat-labeled "unhealthy." The bread is eaten to avoid eating fat. Once you've deleted fat you've also deleted good protein for it usually goes together. What's left? Only carb and people eat plenty of it as they're hungry all the time from elevated insulin. They're eating "healthy" while getting fatter but never put the two together. The church ladies bake the "holy" bread while the starch seeps through the pores with white pasty chalk. The farmer diet fills the body with cement as the protein needs remain unmet and the lack of adequate fat results in constant hunger. The agricultural revolution then and now has debased mankind in body, brain size and certainly happiness as evinced by the crime wave and broken families. So many "health" books extol fruits and grains as if it's an established fact and the AMA continues to cave-in to pressure. Faced with so many contradictions from their constantly changing "food pyramids" the meds deal with the discrepancies by changing it yet again, saying "everyone is different, we all have different needs." Hah! This is not science—this is covering tracks while still trying to appear smart. They just don't know what is happening, and won't know until they eat crow and agree they were wrong by going along with the fat-phobic throng.

If you like carbs so much how about a fig-fast? Here you have maximum cleansing efficiency—it eliminates mucus at a rate of 30 so that the stomach completely cleans out and hunger is completely reduced.   You'll find yourself eating less each day as your body becomes very fit, streamlined and vital. On my last fig-fast I was so amazed at how few figs I needed. The first day I ate a dozen before noon and on the fourth day I could only eat one. I lost all interest in food as the gut became cleaner. This high-carb solution to bakery cravings will surely work for you as a temporary reversal from fat-fasting.

THRIFTY GENE

The human race has surely declined and this can be seen by comparing how they looked in centuries past compared to the disheveled, fat, lopsided specimens we see today.   What causes trouble about the high-carb diet is the thrifty gene: the genetic code passed on from prehistory allowing better survival despite hunger and privation. After periodic famines, natural selection eliminated the weak and left a population who could biochemically squeeze calories out of the food at hand and store it efficiently as fat until needed again. After each meal insulin is called into action and we end up storing too much fat. As the farmer diet keeps insulin high we retain water leading to high blood pressure. Then with insulin there is   increased cholesterol-production causing damage to the arteries--atherosclerosis and heart disease. What did the degeneration of mankind's health do? It evoked more adaptation through the thrifty gene. Man packs on fat as a mal-adaptation to mass diseased (though "advanced" and "wealthy") conditions.

THE FORBIDDEN FOOD IS SEEDS

Seed-grasses like wheat are only 10% water as is the bread they create. This reproductive food substance stimulates passionate feelings in man making him uncontrollably generative--they are aphrodisiac-stimulants creating pugnacity. It's not the meat-eaters who are passionate and pugnacious--it's the bread-eaters. This "passion" for seeds is why the bread and starch are very addicting so they are pumped up as "good" for the "protein" and "roughage" for elimination. But one look at the everyday bread-eater reveals he is not eliminating like he should while the meat-eater who hasn't "enough roughage" looks streamlined and thin. They want the bread to create the very roughage they need to evacuate so they can feel they are making progress. Once one sees how he is stuffed with starch and gives it all up in favor of his prehistoric diet his life changes drastically. It is not fat which encrusts and constipates the system—especially with nuts filled with fiber and colon-happy fat--but rather bread, rice and cereals. There is evacuation--but the tissues remain dry and caked (the "white" man). It is debatable whether cooked food is bad (new science shows it is good as it quickens digestion and thus releases energy to the brain) but machine-concentration of foods is far worse. Seeds are the most concentrated foods in nature, as are legumes and cereals. Such seeds are 60% starch and other non-water-soluble substances that cannot be assimilated and are a tremendous burden on the body.

SEEDS AND WATER: THE WHOLE WORLD
Stuffed with Starch

Like flour paste these substances of seed water and salt (and yeast) is the simple basic diet of most on the earth. After eating them one always thirsts for water, filling out the cells and flesh with toxic waste matter causing "cell burnout" from the combustion of concentrated food. Then one is waterlogged with dead water to keep toxic (salt uric acid) below a strong irritation point. The reproductive part of these plants collect toxic waste matter for elimination so they are saturated with toxins of chemical sprays and fertilizers. So much for starchy grains and legumes.

NO FAT SUBSTITUTES

Only fat restores the natural water balance to body cells avoiding the wrinkles marking old age. It cannot be done by simply adding water to a starchy grain or legume. The calcium in grains and legumes is inorganic, filling the body with dead calcareous deposits collecting in kidneys and gall bladder to form stones and arthritis. Why can't fruits and vegetables restore moisture and then eliminate wrinkles? Because you need protein and fat to give the structure and glow to cells. The older fruitarian is a mass of dry wrinkles having gone without fat. Meat substitutes (seed-proteins the vegetarians use) tear down the body as fast as they build, clogging the system with mucus. Rather than building strong teeth and bones they decalcify the organic calcium. There's no getting around it--you must eat fat and there are no substitutes. To become strong and healthy you must re-achieve your prehistoric status as the hunter.

PUGNACITY

It is said that meat-eaters are "pugnacious". Not so—in the absence of dietary carb they are very happy people. Lovewisdom noticed it's the vegetarians who reveal murderous impulses (against meat-eaters). The vegetarian diet getting "plenty of protein" from beans, grains and seeds gets belligerent as those seed products filling the cells are tissue-irritants. Institutionalized vegetarians living on much heavy seed protein (legumes, grains, wheat germ) are usually schizophrenics. Many vegans become hateful against someone who eats meat. Often the eccentricity of "saints and sages" becomes queer pugnacity when they go starchy vegan. Often the female vegan become "queen guru" to whom everyone runs for advice. She boasts of her recipes using millet and buckwheat and is a walking encyclopedia about veganism. But cross her and she gets cross—the vegan queen bee is often the worst gossip, raising her eyebrow against anyone eating fauna as she cajoles sides against the gypsy hunter-gatherer outcast. Bread is also the seed used by the religious saints who must keep their passions in line by strongly religious feelings and forced "loving thoughts" toward others. The meat-eater is just happy because he is as he should be.

VEGETARIAN TRENDS

"Trends in meat-eating and vegetarian" statistics on the internet reveal the whole world is progressing more towards vegetarianism. Meat-eaters are becoming more rare and often attacked by these growing trends. This is a very interesting development in history (and so sad as fat is replaced by starch) as obesity becomes the predominant pasty look. Take a look at old pictures from the frontier days--the men existing on eggs for breakfast and beef for dinner were tall, thin and handsome until late in life. These old pictures reveal they all looked like Paul Newman. Or look at the old movie moguls--the men were dark and handsome in shiny luster. People had style. The women in the fifties (for the most part) kept themselves like Nancy Reagan: trim, fit and happy (despite what the feminists say). These were the days of meat-eating without shame--it was a matter of course or many courses. Take a look around at the disheveled, fat, sloppy Joe's wearing wrinkled ill-fitting clothes with ring-around-the-collar from the constant-crud-coming-through, and no one cares--they don't have the energy to care.

Starches are the most concentrated foods.   Like flour paste, thirst is created and water-logged toxic waste is crammed into the cells.   The result is indigestion, pain and heartburn. Meat-substitute proteins tear down and clog the body. Rather than building strong teeth and bones they de-calcify and fill the body with inorganic calcium: tissue deposits in man who begins to resemble a leopard. These "dry proteins" generate uric acid throughout the muscles causing rheumatism and arthritis. The high protein in grains, cereals and legumes creates a violent mucus-inundated immuno-suppression. Only fruit, fat and high-water meat (75% H20) restores the correct water balance to cells to avoid wrinkles. Now nuts too are dry but they are paleo and also filled with fat—we've adapted. But not so with dry cereals that need to be drenched with liquid.   Vegetarians with that "leopard look" can be violent: warriors like Hitler and Mussolini were belligerent, ferocious, aggressive and warlike-and vegetarian. The fauna won't make you sick--it's the cereals, rice and breads called "good" and "healthy" which will make you "nutty."

25

SWEET-TEETH

Fruitarian Tooth Decay,
Constriction, Bloat and Anger

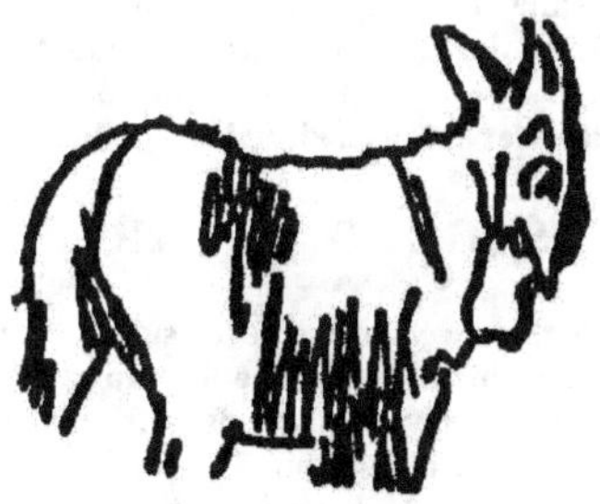

As a fruitarian for twenty years I had various maladies but the most hideous was my teeth crumbling and falling out. It wasn't until I read beyondveg.com that I saw how my deficiency symptoms matched exactly that of other 20-year fruitarians.   The fruitarian fantasy takes over the mind and soul as it beckons one to another world--a separate reality from the mass. It seems so ethereal, so spiritual, so youthful and joyous. I must say that for two decades no one could talk me out of it—I even argued with the dentist as he was restoring my teeth. So possessed was I with this idea that I became a completely different person under a different name.   Many fruitarians are outsiders or post-hippies citing so-called science (e.g. that apes or original man was fruitarian) as karmic law. And this "neo-hippie utopianism" or "quasi fascistic purism" gainsays anyone speaking out against the "accepted" party line.

THE FAT-FAMISHED BRAIN AND SUGAR DRAIN

It took much ill health to finally smash the matrix in my head and accept that animal fat was the only way to recover balance. Fat-famished in the brain, as I look back I seemed insane. And then to eat sugar as substitute, I was lucky I didn't end in institute. By eating a daily fat breakfast then fasting to the next day, the fat pockets from continuous insulin elevation disappeared while the dry skin from lack of fat smoothed out to moistness. The all-day eating of fruit sugar from constant cravings and hunger disappeared to be replaced by complete appetite suppression after only one protein meal. My emotions healed: Change the metabolism and you've changed the person.

BREAD: CRAVE THE GRAVE

The cravings for breads, sugars and fruity snacks is pandemic in America. As bread cleans out eating more bread stops the sick feelings of the cleansing process so he "feels better" and keeps eating it thinking it is "good".   These are the foods Americans binge on, not fauna, but later on the feelings are sleepy, stupid, distended, constricted, bloated. But one feels so good eating fat (an energizer) that soon his tastes all change, no more bakery and bread-deranged. You'll prefer this true human happiness above all else, for as the sweets or starch sock the system into storage one's body becomes filled with ugly protuberances--bags and sags. The body loses logic while in storage mode--the opposite to the slim, streamlined and svelte designed by God to finish the job. You need to conduct the creative act through your veins-- this is your spirit catalyzed through dietary fat. Be a magnetic pole. Do your job in perfect coordination as dietary fat acts as a electrical conduit. Fat means spirit--let it flow!

FAT IS GOOD SUGAR IS BAD

The subject of this chapter is the effects of too much sugar. People think fat is the culprit of all disease. Not so--it is sugar which excites the liver to make its own cholesterol: Fruit-eaters may be filled with it though they eat no foods containing it. In 70% of our childhoods we had totally unnatural lives as we indiscriminately ate so much sugar and starch and the result is a nation of fat people. People looked so much better mid-century when families sat down to three balanced meat meals with butter, lard, cheese, cream and many courses of meat with no eating in between. Most people stayed trim and fit much longer than the gargantuan unnatural bodies we see today starting in childhood.

INSULIN CRAVINGS

This constant elevation of insulin creates lowered blood sugar (we're always hungry); a shift into storage mode (we lay on fat); conversion of sugar and protein to fat (everything we eat makes us fat); a removal of fat from the blood which is then put into fat cells (landing on the hips, thighs, guts, upper arms and legs); an increase in cholesterol, water and salt-retention by the   kidneys (we become puffy and peevish); growth of arterial cells (the beginnings of closed arteries so blood pressure is raised) and the use of glucose for energy (rather than using our own fat for energy-ketosis-which is what we want for slimness and perfect health).

We may have started life on a balanced diet but in most cases it became unbalanced by our teen years when taste usually swerves to carbs. Now sugar and starch formed the bulk of what was eaten: beans, breads and baked goods, cakes and candies, pasta, rice, fried potatoes, popcorn, "pop-tarts" and other man-made inventions. Illogical food cravings typify this state in which hunger is never satiated while the gut expands into bulk fullness. One finishes a big dinner only to be hungry later. Cravings, hunger, fatigue and bad moods indicate carb metabolism is abnormal. Only a diet low in carbs and high in fat and protein brings recovery and satisfaction in which is great joy.

ENTER FRUITARIANISM

70% of us have IR this hyper-insulin condition. So now we become excited over fruitarianism. Wow! What a spiritual life: we can all see it, we recognize it from the primordial depths of consciousness to the beginning of the Garden of Eden. And so we dig into the sweet fruit happily thinking we will now become supermen and gods on earth only to find that our abdomens are distended (many develop Candida), that we have mean morose moods and that the cravings never cease. Many young fruitarians polish off a box of dates (no sweat these sweets) only to meet a new craving for the very starchy-gluey-fleshy morsels of the SAD culture-food they disdain. The common result: recurrent closet binges. If 70% of us have this deranged metabolism, for 70% of us the only cure is lowcarb dieting which automatically means fat and protein. Many fruitarianism experience diabetes-like symptoms: excess urination, frequent thirst, mood swings, intermittent blurred vision, pains in extremities (hands and feet) and frequent fatigue (which they call "detox") from consuming grossly excessive carbs given the common level of insulin resistance.

CANDIDA

Too-much sugar in the diet can often lead to the outgrowth of candida, a yeast. Systemic yeast infection--when candida is all through the body, organs and tissues--develops from suppressed immunity from protein and fat deficiency. The result is lethargy, fatigue, depression, headaches, constipation, mental sluggishness and slurred speech, gas in the lower abdomen, bloating, ab-pain, brain fog, distention and tremendous breathing problems. Most A.I.D.s, cancer and Environmental Illness patients have it and I certainly did. (However my fat-fasting regime boosted immunity so that now I can eat even figs, raisins or pineapple each morning and it is kept within bounds.) Atkins says one-third of his patients have it and once they do secondary allergies arise to other common foods like grains (corn, wheat, rye, oats), soy, milk, cheese, eggs, brewers and bakers yeast, the nightshades (potato, tomato, eggplant), coffee, citrus, dairy, shellfish, beef, chicken, onions, peppers, spices, mushrooms. In these early days when I was still protein-deficient I found I was allergic to eggs the indicator being bloated and painful legs. The worst the withdrawal the better you will now feel. These were the foods you loved and gave you a slight lift then let you way down and out all due to candida from starch and sugar.

ADAPTATION TO MEAT

There is so much evidence (beyondveg.com) that humans have always eaten and are perfectly adapted to eating meat. For a hypersensitive with food allergies meat may be the only thing they can eat. Like the heme iron receptor sites on the intestines for example which absorb iron from meat and thus are clear evidence of adaptation to meat-eating. Also our B-12 needs are only found in animal foods.   For any mammal animal foods are easier than plant foods to digest for structural (cell wall) reasons. Many plant foods inhibit digestion due to evolutionary dependence on animal foods for nutrients like iron zinc and animal protein. This carnivore-connection--the human as hunter--explains the high incidence of diabetes-like symptoms and failure rates among fruitarians. Most people are not genetically adapted to a diet in which 75% of calories come from sugar! Fruitarians have frequent mood swings and fatigue from the abnormal elevation of insulin. Here is where genetic evolution is slowly influencing nutritional knowledge: sugar (constant fruit) and seeds (beans and grains) are non-evolutionary foods creating health risks both biochemically and   genetically but especially by suppressing the immune system.

SYMPTOMS OF FAILURE TO THRIVE

One does well on all-fruit for months or a year but then there is a decline--a lack of energy, fatigue and hunger all the time. In some we see B-12 deficiency, lost sex drive, hyperactivity and respiratory problems.   These "pure diets" show initial improvement followed by long-term decline. It feels so good at first they can't believe it will go sour. Detox does feel good but over long-term it extracts sufficient nutrition and causes "deficiency-disease" syndromes which are subtle and slowly debilitating.   Billings calls this the "lulling effect of imperceptibility" in a decline in health: Because the victim doesn't want to believe it is happening he is lulled into false security and his deficiency symptoms make him think he needs more detox. The fruitarian is extremely anti-authority so won't believe his family and friends while being completely hypnotized by the detox matrix which he sees with complete certitude to be the whole point to disease vs. health. (It's only half the point—fat-rebuilding and nourishment is the other.) Because initial results make him feel all problems are signs of detox, emotional "certainty" shuts down reason.

SALVATION VIA INTERNET

Had I not come upon Tom Billing's site beyondveg.com I would have fruitlessly continued in my failure to thrive for the fruitarian cannot ascertain what's gone wrong and gets only pat answers from the leaders and magazines. It's a "calories paradox" of eating like a horse but feeling hungry all the time. Naturally they become tempted by "illegal" foods and there is often periodic binging. The "sufficiency" of fruit-only is a myth of the party-line: "truths" that simply aren't so. Only after escaping dogma and restoring health can he put practical results before dogma. Billings makes other good points:

Via the internet we can come to grips with reality as we bypass party line leaders and compare notes. Ah-ha: we see increasing evidence that private reality is at odds with the public face of veganism as long-term "raw" failures are becoming widely acknowledged. We begin to see how dogma superceded compassion for when the fruit diet fails people are blamed.   We can also see how idealism encourages junk science to get converts to "uncritically accept or creatively interpret" facts with little diligence. This is the psychology of denial coming from exclusive reliance on case studies with no evidence but hearsay. People only study what they think to look for so "failure to thrive" and deficiencies are not "seen" and since those discussing it risk moral ostracism former vegans are not heard or believed. Studies of paleopathology show marked longevity and health of paleo hunters vs. Neolithic farmers based on fossil bone analysis. Since "natural" fruit diets are refuted by this evidence the fruit-gurus attack the idea of micro-evolution of diet itself.

MODERN PALEO RESEARCH

The late role of grains and legumes ("evolutionary discordance") show health risks but aren't studied because few medical researchers see the relevance of late role in evolution. Society for 25 years has seen high-carb as good and high-protein as dangerous. Yet evolutionary research strongly indicates that high protein and low carb is the correct macronutrient ratio with great effects on the heart. Initially they thought high-protein brought calcium excretion and osteoporosis yet Paleolithic fossil bones show excellent skeletal status. New paleo-scientists are now rethinking the effects of fat since hunter-gatherers ate at least 50% animal food and especially the fat of the animal. Metabolic evidence shows man is like cats: completely dependent on nutrients in animal fats that are not easily synthesized from plant foods. Let me ask you a simple question: if you gave a dog or cat a choice between meat or some fruit or vegetable which one would he take? Well modern science shows man has much the same physiological needs. Humans have been eating meat since their beginning with no evidence of a strict fruitarian society as hunter-gathering societies ate meat and no tribes were totally vegan let alone fruitarian.

STRAW MAN ARGUMENTS

"Morphology and physiology intertwined: morphological markers like body size and shape are regulated by hormones (physiology). Morphological evolution is driven by physiological evolution"(Billings). Size and shape are regulated by hormones like insulin and glucagons. Look around to the bulbous size and shape today--welcome to the 21st century. The human is meant to be beautiful and thin by the correct diet and the elevation of glucagons from high fat and low carb alternating with the constant detox (cleansing effects) of the fruit and daily fasting. Moreover humans are not built to collect fruit--only four-footed apes are. Continuous fruit-eating is not feasible for hunter-gatherers. An increase in brain and a decrease in gut size is possible only via an increase in DQ-dietary quality from fat with fruit.

FROM THE BEGINNING: RECAP

The whole fruitarian argument is outdated through recent science: (1) the fruitarian picture of a Garden of Eden and (2) the "comparative anatomy" argument (i.e. apes as fruitarians) which is now shown false through modern studies of apes who as frugi-faunivores eat meat in the form of insects. The apes studies themselves says Billings are "irrelevant given the direct evolutionary data on the early human diet now available." The natural hygiene model is purely subjective. These raw-food vegetarian diets can get real results in the short term but lead to tragic deficiencies in the long-term since they restrict the evolutionary diet. "The restriction of real needs in pursuit of 'purity' often leads to physical collapse and a vicious cycle of circular mental logic: imbalance combines with fanaticism to trap the dense believer indefinitely.

Now the spirit expressly says that in latter times some will depart from the faith giving heed to deceiving spirits and doctrines of demons speaking lies in hypocrisy having their own conscience seared with a hot iron. Forbidding to marry and commanding to abstain from foods which God created to be received with thanksgiving by those who believe and know the truth. For every creature of God is good and nothing is to be refused if it is received with Thanksgiving for it is sanctified by the word of God and prayer. Timothy 1: 4

FFF Recipes

These are my recipes for the frugi-fatarian-fastarian
Lifestyle and I hope you enjoy them too.

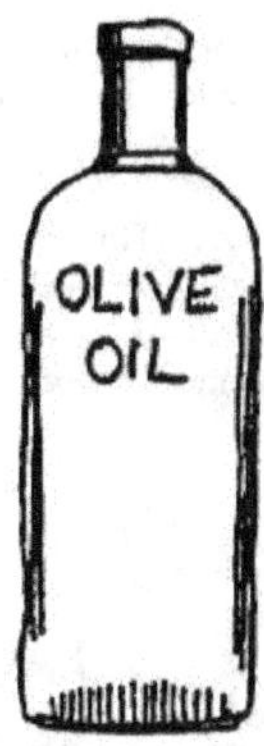

The fruit diet which is all juicy or dried fruit and avocados. The higher paleo
diet is fruit, fat (nuts, cheese, avocados) and occasional greens. The lacto-
fruitarian diet is fruit and dairy. The paleo-diet is low carb salads, omelets or
fish. All diets are combined with

THE DAILY FAST

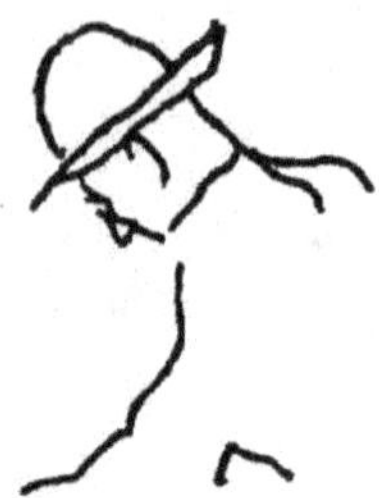

for bliss, God's kiss and a perfect day with nothing amiss. Though we may begin the fast with a feast, with each day we see that the fast IS the feast (where joy never ceased as our health has increased).

Fatarian Law: Wait on hour for satiety. Then don't eat past noon--and oh how you'll swoon, for the aft-fast is your Glory Church. RX: Breakfast: fruit or juice. Lunch: the frugi-fat recipes below. Then just skip dinner, and do that every single day. For the cheese recipes get the LITTLE DIPPER warmer, the only kitchen appliance you'll ever need.

DIETS

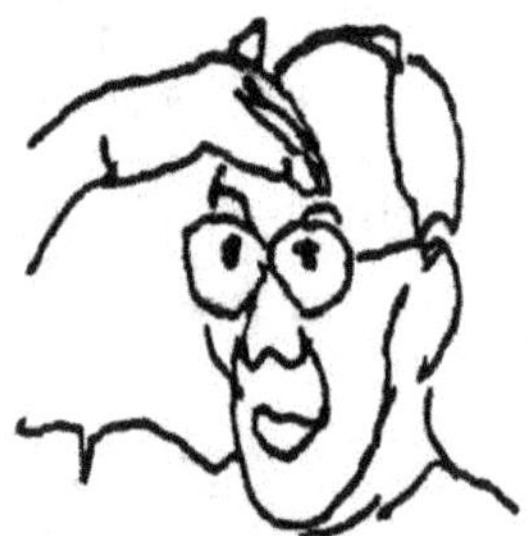

Rastafarian Fruitarianism
Fish with non-sweet fruit salads, squash and eggplant (fruits)

Ovo-Lacto Fruitarianism
Eggs and or dairy with fruits (sweet or non-sweet)

Lacto-Fruitarian
Cheese and Fruit Diet

Frugi-Nutbutterarianism (Spoon Theory)
Fruit and Frugal Nutbutter Fasting with Weekly Fauna

SHOPPING

Fill your home with good things with longevity in bulk: good quality cheeses aged naturally (not cheap cheeses with bacteria added), olive oil, raisins, prunes, figs, nuts, olives, tomato paste, canned applesauce or pineapple chunks in their own juice (no sugar), garlic powder, seasonings (Italian or Indian most healing), lemon juice, green apples, purified water and good coffee—and fresh produce for your Red Salads and fruit snacks. Regarding veggies, this diet is not rabbit food but delicious fruit and fat for the best health which is thin, not fat. Now you'll be shiny and elastic, like a cat.

NEW WAY TO EAT:
Without Starch, No Need for so Much Water

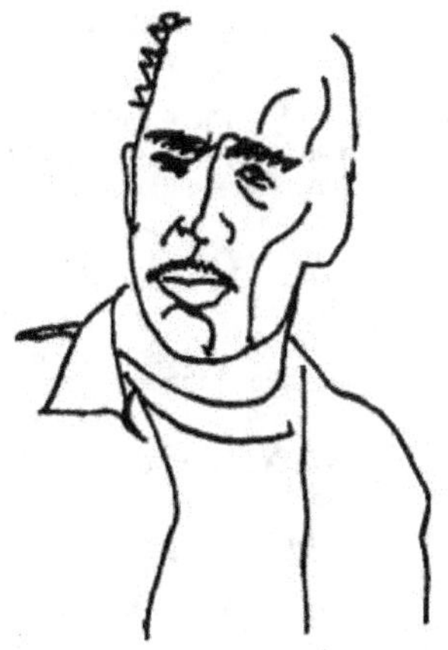

EARLY CALIFORNIA

I live in the California desert which is "Mestizo"--a combination of Spanish and Indian influences. I have read every book written on the old Spanish Missions, the ranchos, the Indian tribes here the food and the fashions. What a history! I love my environment and as I walk around in the barren desert I see arrowheads on the ground, massive amounts of pottery coming up from the deep earth, old burial grounds and ritual circles. Fashion: Early California designs and clothes painting. Food: See below (Latin minus the tortillas, pasta, rice and beans).

The Fat-fruitarian-fastarian diet is composed of fruit (sweet or non-sweet) and FAT from fruits, nuts and fauna (animal protein and fat). With these recipes the feeling of rare satiety will enable you to go long periods in a fun fabulous fast. You will no longer dream of food or crave it, just enjoy it immensely (but the fast even more). On cooking: the longer your doughless pizza warms the more flavorful and appetite suppressing. Tomato or paste, the juices and spices form a film or delicious crust of pure flavorful fat, and you'll be full (just like that). I warm the doughless pizza sometimes overnight. After eating fat-flavorful foods such as the recipes below there is "full" satiety, because the less you eat and the more the fat content the more KETOTIC (i.e. appetite-suppressing, fat-burning and energy-evoking). Once you get going, just read this book --the insights will be flowing as you're coming into the "knowing

FFF MAINSTAYS

RED SALAD

Slice tomatoes and red bell peppers with lemon juice, olive oil and avocado. Optional: leaves and cucumber. An exhilarating, delicious blood stimulant and great for the daily meal of red genius. Optional: cheese or fish.

TOMAVO

In blender: 2 tomatoes, 2 avocados, ,lemon juice. This is great for cancer victims who can't eat without pain--just a little mild tomavo in the morning and they can happily fast all day.

HEAVENLY GUACAMOLE

In blender: two lg. avocado or 4 small, 2 tomatoes, one jalapeno, 3 cloves garlic, bunch cilantro, tab. olive oil. Enjoy your delicious fat-fasting vacation beginning with this guacamole and then eat low carb in restaurants.

SALSA

I like mine extra hot but this is mild. In blender: 3 tomatoes, bunch cilantro,1 jalapeno, juice of lime, 2 cloves garlic. Lay down and feel the implosive cleansing action of salsa go to work—there is no faster cleanser. Optional: add greens like green onions. For fruitarian salsa, delete the onions and garlic and add avocado for guacamole.

GREEN GODDESS

In blender: two avocados, lemon juice, three green onions and three garlic cloves. Delicious as dip with raw celery.

FAT SALAD

Put in bowl: can black olives, handful cashews, cheese slivers, generous lemon and olive oil (optional: fish and/or cherry tomatoes).

AVOCADO RECIPES

ALL FATS ARE A FIND: THEY GIVE YOU A SHINE

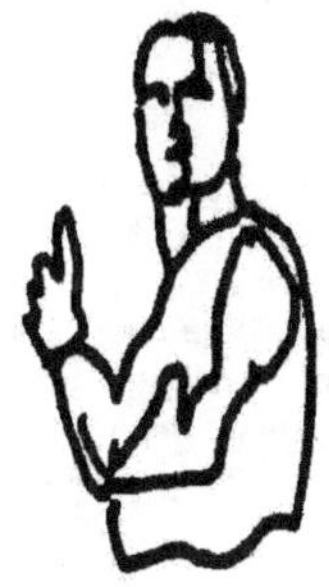

In blender or cut up on plate:

PINAVO: Pineapple chunks with avocado

TOMAVO: sliced tomato and avocado with lemon

CUCAVO: sliced cucumber with avocado and lime

CITAVO: citrus sliced with avocado

LIMAVO: lime, avocado and jalapeno in blender

BELLAVO: red bells/avocado sliced with lemon juice/olive oil, cilantro

GREENAVO: avocado, lemon juice, garlic cloves in blender

AVOCADO SOUP (cold): blend avos with green onion, lemon, tomato and for something different a clove of garlic and sour cream

DIVINE DESSERTS

From the Desert Holy Lands:
Raisins and Nuts

TRAIL MIX FAST

Karen: My mother loves to nibble and eats candy all day. She refuses fruit as "health food" but has been snacking on Planter's cashews for years. How can I transition her to your diet?"

What this calls for is a TRAIL MIX FAST: Give her unlimited bowls of raisins and cashews together. The raisins clean the gut (reason for abnormal hunger-- dirty gut) while the nuts roto-rooter it all out. It is so delicious and like everything else about this diet, her cravings will taper off and she'll eat far less with time. If she craves a little more while on restriction, just a piece of cheese. This blend is more like candy but with twice the cleansing action of juicy fruit, combined with the colon-happy fatty nuts which are pure evacuative action.

NUT-BUTTER FASTING
Spoon Theory

Karen, What is a nut-butter fast? When eating, enjoy fruits and salmon once a week. When fasting, take a couple tablespoons of nut butter in the morning then fast all day. Finally free of hunger, you'll learn to see things a whole new way. WARNING: 5% have fatal peanut allergies and I think it's because it's not a nut it's a legume—a bean! That's not keen but nut-butters are a cool tool to stop being an eating fool for cravings can be cruel).. With nutbutter fasting (spoon theory) you overcome food addiction and become the master not the mule. Buy chunky no-salt natural nut butter and never overdo—the point is a spoon or two (not more than a few) and just watch as your skin becomes like dew! For the ex-glutton to achieve fastarian consciousness there is no other way—just learn how to enjoy the day this way, with only nutbutters and the ray. The nut butter is only 7 carbs for two tabs, and it's very evacuative. I buy a 35-pound barrel of chunky no-salt each month for myself and four dogs.

Fiestas

This is lowcarb with protein. These recipes are for special occasions or those allergic to nuts. We fast, we feast—but we stick to foods from the FFF model at least. I recommend sweet or non-sweet Greek fruit salads and weekly salmon but these are my other recipes using cheese, fish and eggs:

DOUGHLESS PIZZA
(Italian Fat Fast)

FOR PEOPLE ON THE GO : NO TIME FOR SHOW

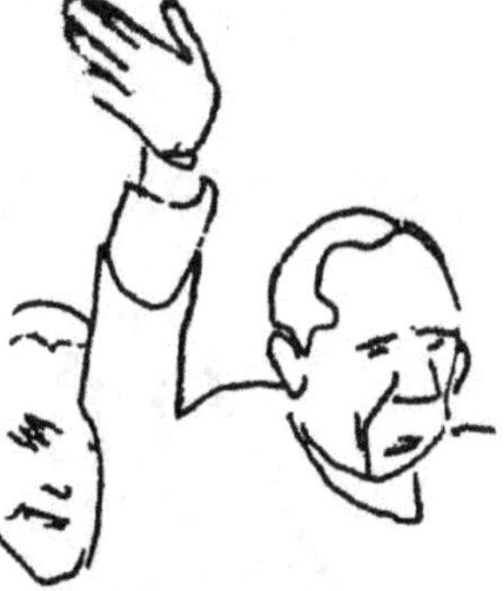

Slice zuchini, tomato and white onion. Put a little cheese in the wafflizer and add the sliced fruit. Put parmasan on top and close the wafflizer, cook for five minutes or until brown on both sides. Doughless pizza recipe 2: Get a tiny crock pot ("little dipper") warmer—essential for fatarians. Plan to eat in one hour after the cheese melts in with olive oil, garlic powder, a little tomato paste or sliced tomatoes, cashews and black olives. The fattier, the better—the richer, the more it suits this theory to the letter. The other meal should be just raisins or figs and nuts. Caution: avoid cheeses like low fat mozzarella, some swiss or the spreadables—they contain starch substitutes or corn starch (bad). Also read labels on juices: things like "apple cocktail" contains cornstarch. When this theory says "fat" it's referring to animal fat—fauna—not vegetable oil which will kill you.

CHILI RELLENO

How I always loved chile rellenos! Try chilli relleno casseroles. Here's my rendition: dice one tomato and half green or red peppers. Put in warmer with jack cheese and some cashews. Melt for one-two hours, enjoy. Wow—right now this is my favorite special week-end chows preceding the day fast.

CRUMBS

Cook doughless pizza in the warmer for 8-10 hours. The tomato paste forms a delicious dark crust—this slow and long-cooked zero-carb pizza is a must. Put in container and eat a few crumbs when hungry. You won't believe how delicious and satisfying it is being a "crumb-eater".

☐☐ITALIANO MARIA

Put plenty of olive oil in pan—never fear the fat. Add garlic powder, Italian seasonings and a little parmesan cheese. Lay in sliced tomatoes in the pan. Slice cheese on top—swiss or mozzarella. Let cook until crispy on bottom with delicious tomato sauce from the cooked tomatoes. The more tomatoes you use the better. It's low in carbs though filled with the most cleansing fruit and herbs.

Variations:

Eggplant/ Zucchini Parmesan
Add sliced eggplant or zucchini to the above

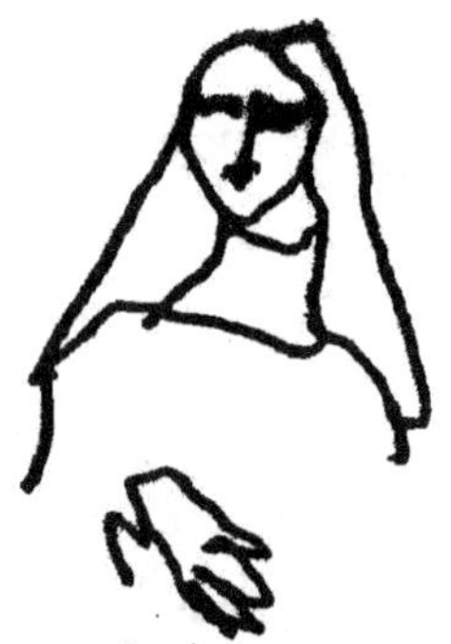

Italian Bell-Melt

Put Italian and garlic seasonings in a pan with much olive oil. Slice bell peppers (all colors) into the pan, cover with tomatoes and cheese. Can be broiled but you won't have the sauce and you can also substitute with tomato paste (Springfield has no salt).

Red Delicious

Wonderful with guacamole. Saute minced garlic in olive oil in pan. Cover with tomato slices and after ten minutes lay in sliced red cabbage on top—fry or broil until there's a delicious red gravy.

CHAMPION GUIDES

Tomato Melt

Put plenty of olive oil in pan—never fear the fat. Add garlic powder,
Italian seasonings and a little parmesan cheese. Lay in sliced
tomatoes in the pan. Slice cheese on top—swiss or mozzarella. Let
cook until crispy on bottom with delicious tomato sauce from the
cooked tomatoes. The more tomatoes you use the better. It's low in
carbs though filled with the most cleansing fruit and herbs.

Stewed Red Au Gratin

In Little Dipper dice one or two tomatoes with Italian seasonings
and garlic powder with your cheese, cashews and olive oil. Let
tomatoes make a rich red gravy after two hours warming. Optional:
add sliced red bells, green onions or zucchini as per taste. Great
after pineapple.

Cucavo Maria

In blender: juice of one lime, three avocados, one cucumber, one
tomato, two jalapenos, some cilantro. Enjoy the delightfully
different, cool and fresh taste of this guacamole. The low-sugar
cucumber is excellent for skin, nails, hair and teeth and a wonderful
alkalinizer.

Cheese Omelet

Put olive oil or butter in frying pan. Add minced onion and garlic
powder. Add diced bell peppers or zucchini. Beat three eggs and
pour in the pan with cheese on top. Fold omelet and cook on both
sides

Spanish Omelet

Add salsa to the cheese omelet and serve with guacamole

Fruit Cheese Cake

Pineapple cheesecake is my one meal a day. Cheese eaten with apples is also
good (thus breaking all food combining rules). Warm the cheese in the
warmer with diced apples or pineapple (optional: raisins and nuts). Warm
for two hours, cut like quiche. Tastes like apple pie with cheese.

Apple Raisin Nut Coffee Cake

Slice granny smith apples into pan with butter, raisins and cashews. Add cinnamon and cheese for frugi-fatarian bliss and for something a little different, add doughless pizza crumbs.

RASTAFARIAN

Means FISH for your one meal a day:

Lemon Cashew Tuna

This you'll love. In Little Dipper put olive oil, a LOT of fresh lemon juice (I use the juice of two lemons), cashews and a can of albacore with ½ lb cheese. Melt it all together, and eat bites when hungry. The lemon lends a delightful tang.

Cashew Albacore Melt

Put albacore, cheese and cashews with a lot of olive oil in a pan. Cook until a little brown (crispy) on the bottom. Put it in the frig and take small bites when hungry. A 6 oz can of albacore tuna should last you two days with happy appetite suppression. You can use fish or cheese with these everyday recipes below.

Manhattan Fish/Cheese Stew

Dice 2-3 tomatoes in Little Dipper with olive oil, garlic powder, Italian seasonings, tuna or salmon as per taste, cheese, cashews. Optional: zucchini, another non-sweet fruit, Warm two hours. Great after a cup of diced pineapple.

Salmon Salad

Put 6 oz salmon in bowl and add many cashews, mucho lemon juice and olive oil. Enjoy.

Cheese and Fish Omelet

Put much olive oil in pan, add cheese, 6 oz. fish and some cashews (diced onion optional). Whip up three eggs and add to pan when cheese is melted. Scramble or make omelet.

Tuna Salad

In a bowl: one-half minced onion, one-half head lettuce shredded fine, cilantro, diced cucumber, bell pepper and black olive (optional). Put in a can of tuna and herb salt to taste. Add lemon and olive oil and enjoy this delicious meal along with the luxurious afternoon as it digests and cleans with the protein, leaves and elevation of glucagons.

Tuna Melt

Put cut string beans (canned, frozen or fresh) in little dipper with olive oil, lemon juice, canned salmon or tuna, cashews and cheese to taste. Warm one-two hours and add sour cream if you like.

Rastafarian Red Salad

Add tuna or white fish to the Red Salad Recipe. Food addicts tortured by cravings report complete satisfaction after one daily fish salad or omelet meal—the cravings are gone and they lose weight.

Rastafarian Red Delicious

Add tuna or white fish to the Red Delicious recipe. White fish doesn't create mucus or acid like other meats

Salmon Cheese Omelet with Cashews

Add a 6-oz fresh salmon and cashews to the omelet above, or take on the side with a little lemon juice and olive oil cooked in it.

SCAVENGERS

In all flavors, they do you no favors!

I'd avoid all garbage-eaters and cockroaches of the sea (scavengers) if you wish to have perfect health and look your best. I know they are the most delicious--pig, lobster, scallops, oysters, clams, shrimp, crab and catfish to name a few--but if you could see them in the spirit you'd say "pee-ooo". Pork lard does <u>not</u> rule! So don't be a fool, these most common meats are <u>not</u> cool. The pig and the rat are equally unclean. And if you put scallops in a filthy pool, they'll fill with putridity and the pool will be clean--a food like that will not give you sheen. They've been put on the earth to vacuum bacteria so if you eat them you'll get weak (and become a suck-up not a superior man mock-up). So listen up: stick to fauna the Lord said to eat and leave these "delicious filthy morsels" for the mortal's" treat".

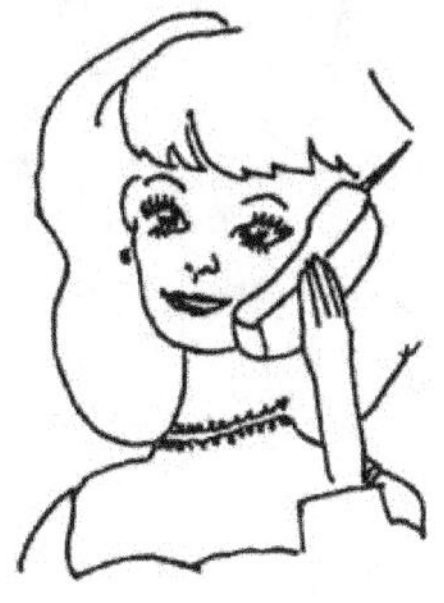

No need to call out. These recipes are far more delicious and you know they're clean (made with someone with sheen who's never mean).   Isn't it nice just to stay home and enjoy it like Rome?

NOW, FAST

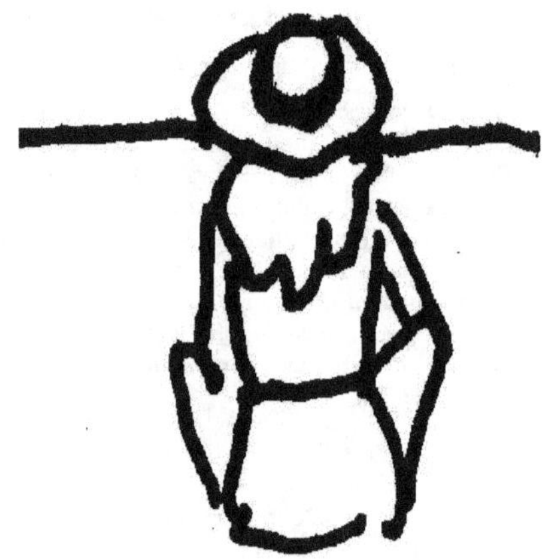

Daily Dog Food (Best Friend) Recipes

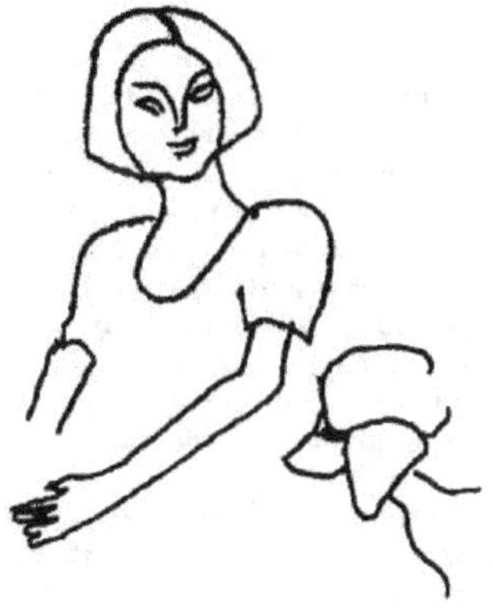

"BARF" DIET

(Bones and Raw Food)

For humans, dogs and cats, grains are bad and vegetables are secondary. Here are two known methods, and one transition:

1. RMB'S-ONLY

No More Doggie Odor, Dry Fur, Begging or Vets

Dogs have always been called omnivores--but many are beginning to see then as pure carnivores: in the wild they live on raw meat and bones mainly, and any reliance on vegetables is questionable. The BARF DIET (Bones and Raw Food for Dogs) reflects the wolf's diet in the wild. I choose the RMBs (raw meaty bones) because of the sudden difference I've witnessed in my five-pack. The raw chicken bones won't splinter like the cooked so don't worry about that, and dogs (unlike humans) can handle the bacteria in raw chicken meat. An example of a RMB DINNER would be chicken or turkey backs, whole legs and wings, lamb neck bones, beef ribs, sardines or canned mackerel, and organ meat (liver, kidney). For most raw-givers, chicken forms the basis of the raw diet because it's cheap, but essential also are organ meats and chewy (for their teeth) beef ribs. Now your dogs will live a long happy life--watch them come alive because they're finally getting the real thing.

Most raw givers don't believe in the necessity of supplements or vegetables--the main ingredient should be fauna (RMBs)

2. RMB'S WITH VEGGIES AND EGGS

The BARF Diet used for the hypersensitive greyhounds uses equal parts raw veggies and raw meaty bones. You spend a couple hours a month to prepare the meals and put it in your freezer (I recommend getting a 5 cubic freezer from Sears). In the morning you give them their "salad meal" and in the evening, raw meat and bones. <u>Salad am:</u> use a variety but the base is equal parts raw veggies and raw meat blended with raw egg. Pre-ground the meat (e.g. liver), a variety of vegetables, garlic cloves (one per day), collard greens, carrots, raw eggs, raw honey, vinegar, and oil (flaxseed oil, salmon, or fish body oil but flaxseed is the most healthful omega fatty acids). Mix thoroughly in a food processor and place in resealable container (yogurt containers are good). Make a batch to last a couple of weeks, and you're all set. The mixture will give your dog carbs, enzymes, antioxidants, vitamins, minerals, essential fatty acids simulating the wild diet.

Karen: Why don't you believe in raw meat for humans? KK: Because man has adapted to cooked food from the beginning (see beyondveg.com) whereas dogs have not--they <u>need</u> raw meat and bones for their teeth and everything else. Regarding bacteria in raw meat, they have the capacity to deal with bacteria (like the pig) whereas humans don't.

3. RMBs with STEAMED MEAT OR STEWS

Transition to Rawfoodism. Despite the upgrade it's not always easy making the transition-- dogs don't like having their diets changed suddenly: Most all dogs love the raw beef ribs but few like the raw chicken and liver and I refuse to force it on them. So I steamed the liver and chicken but made the majority of their diet the raw beef ribs. Simultaneously they ceased eating any kibble, for just like humans they were finally satisfied with far less of the HQ (higher quality). Having removed the rice and kibble their diet was completely RMBs with some steamed meat. I was delighted to see that each day they needed less food for satiety. For some dogs the transition diet from commercial food might be the broth/stew route: cook five big whole chicken legs in a 20-cup steamer with water and perhaps some diced garlic and carrot. After about 45 minutes its done with in a greasy (good) flavorful sauce. Avoid onions which are toxic for dogs, and remove the cooked bones, which splinter. This delicious meaty broth (pure flavor) filled with grease and meat will satisfy the dogs along with their RMB's each day. If you dog prefers the raw liver or chicken that is better. Chicken and rice is not recommended, for dogs cannot handle grains which lead to allergies.

DOG FOOD COMPANY KILLERS

Disgusting Death Mills

Pet food industries only use ingredients that are unfit for human consumption, making a profit from waste that would otherwise be worthless. Moreover, the preservatives in commercial dog food destroy their kidneys. By the time you see the first symptoms of lassitude it's too late—they are dead within weeks for once the kidneys go there's no possible prevention. These preservatives—six of which are known poisonous carcinogens outlawed in human food—kill millions of pets every single year. These poisons are known to create stomach cancer, spleen cancer, leukemia, major organ failure, immune system collapse, severe allergic reactions, birth defects, blindness, chronic diarrhea, hair loss and behavior problems—and this even refers to foods labeled "chemical and preservative free", as manufacturers don't have to list poisons that they themselves did not add (like from rendering plants). Moreover, rendering plants can use euthanized dogs and cats killed by sodium pentobarbital, or tumors and huge cancerous cysts off of cows and sheep. You fatten their pockets while they kill your dogs.

CAT FOOD HIGHER IN PROTEIN--BUT NOT MUCH

It's Still Half-Carb--Preposterous!

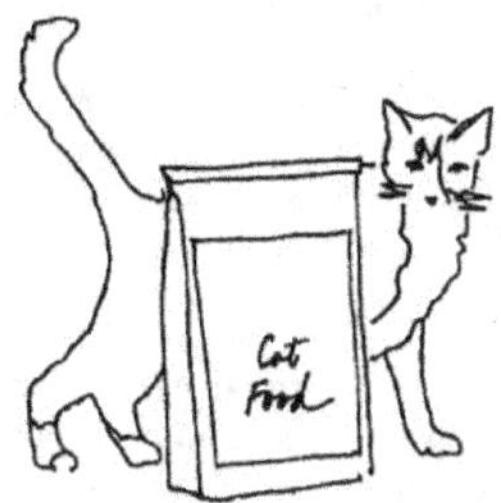

Once they wake-up to the higher protein in cat food while seeing how their dogs love it, they are tempted to give it to them instead of dog food. Cat foods are also dangerous but at least they are higher in protein: since cats are known carnivores and dogs omnivores, dog food companies get away with much higher starch content. But dry cat food is still half carbohydrate, resulting in fat cats. Further, the fat content is from sprayed fats which make both dog and cat love them as a mirage. It would be best to feed cats a high-end cat food which is all protein, and make your dogs food just meat. The dollar difference between starchy food and high-protein meaty food is billions. We all know that dog food has become increasingly starchy over the last couple decades--it began with far more protein--and that may be one reason dogs die around twelve though many cats hit twenty. Research shows that starchy dogs develop clogged arteries in their legs but dogs given pure animal protein remain sleek and energetic with clear arteries (just like humans). Protein is immunoenhancing so they can keep parasites away while starch is immuno-suppressive so dog owners have to pay billions more for pet-meds. it's really sad what's happening to dogs due to naive vets caving into these money hungry industries and fat-phobic public opinion, as most vets are taught nutritional science from pet food companies themselves.

NEVER TRUST BIG CORPS WITH YOUR PETS

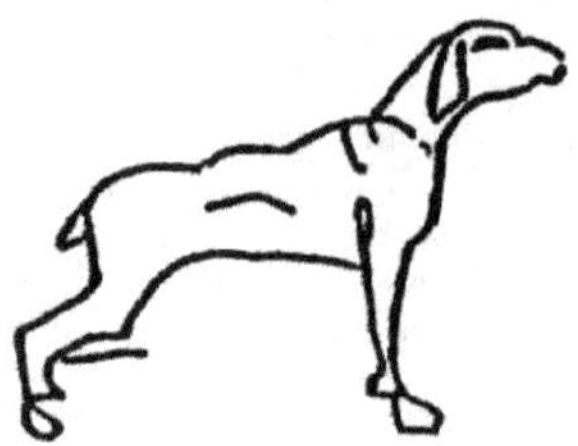

Raw meaty bones make dogs cute, sleek, bouncy and slick. Commercial pet food makes them slow, fatigued, dry and sick.

The pet food industries only use ingredients that are unfit for human consumption. They make a profit from waste that would otherwise be worthless. Meat received from the slaughterhouse is "denatured" by covering it with such poisons as carbolic acid (phenol, a corrosive disinfectant), fuel oil, kerosene--all to prevent human consumption. Also included is disabled, diseased, dead or dying animals. Other rendered items include restaurant grease and leftovers, road kill, euthanized pets complete with flea collars and the green bags in which they are transported, and grocery store items such as old baked goods. So why does your dog come running when you open a new bag? Because that overpowering odor smells like dinner as smelly gluey fat is sprayed directly on the morsels of food. Sticking flavors onto dry morsels tricks pets into eating the food. Now if you skip commercially packed foods completely and feed your pet RMBs he'll eat far less because he is using all of the nutrition he's getting instead of it passing through his body unused.

Your pet is not just an animal, he's a member of your family--in pure innocence he will eat whatever his owner gives him. So take the time to protect him by giving him the true thing: raw meaty bones!

Proclamation!

VEGAN DOGMA FORCED ON DOGS!

Having come from a raw foods background I am very aware of how raw vegetables are being imposed on dogs ("until they eat it") and even poor cats who are pure carnivores. Yes, cats are carnivores and dogs are omnivores but they both do best on animal foods. With low fat diets their immunity is suppressed and they become filled with every parasite. Switching to fauna fat is like an instant transformation as lazy, dry and lackluster dogs became shiny puppies exuberant with new found energy. This should be such a serious matter to all dog and cat lovers. My vegan neighbor forced white rice and raw vegetables on her poor dog who had no personality nor energy whatsoever. When people come to my home they are amazed at these dogs "who are more like people". The vegan will say "but meat makes dogs violent" but I have observed just the opposite to be the case.

LOVE DOGS AS PART OF THE FAMILY

Don't make em eat crap while they see you eating incredibly delicious food! Don't be a meanie and eat your daily meal as a family but no begging later—you're in this together.

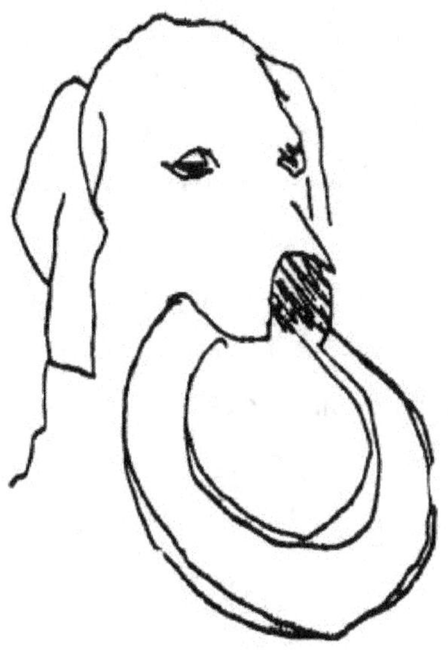

BIBLIOGRAPHY

Aiello and Wheeler in Current Anthropology 1995.

Atkins Robert. *Dr. Atkins New Diet Revolution* Avon Books 1992

Benoit F.et.al. Changes in body composition during Weight reduction in obesity" Arch. Of internal Medicine 63:4 (1965) p 604-612

Billings Tom. Beyondveg.com

Cassidy Claire Ph.D. In *Protein Power* p 401

Cockburn Mummies Diseases and Ancient Cultures in Eades p. 400

Eades Michael and Mary Dan M.D. *Protein Power* 1996 Bantam Books

Graham, Douglas. *Grain Damage: Rethinking the High Starch Diet*

Howard Vernon. No *50 Ways to Escape Cruel People* 1981

James William. *Varieties of Religious Experience* 1858.

Lovewisdom John. "Vitarianism" unpub. Manuscript 1975.

O'Dea Dr. Kerin in *Protein Power* by Eades and Eades p. 46

Schachter Zalman and Ronald Miller. *From Age-ing to Sage-ing* Warner Books 1995.

100 KAREN KELLOCK BOOKS

AFFINITY OR MISERY
AGELESS CORNUCOPIA
AMERICA AWAKE!
AMERICA'S DAFT ERA
ARTS OF PALEO FASTING
AUTOPHAGY ON CHEATERS
BACKSTABBING NEUROTICS
BETRAYAL TRAUMA
BOOMERS AND BROKENNESS
BOOT ON NECK
CHAMPION GUIDES
COMMIE NUTHOUSE
COMMIES
COMMUNIST SPIRIT
CONTAGION OF MADNESS
CONTAGIOUS MADNESS
CULTURE CLASH BASHED
DAFT LEFT
DAILY FASTARIAN
DAM RATS
DIVERSITY IS CRUELTY
E-RACE WHITE
EVIL FREAKS (Beyond Gross)
THE END OR A BEND?
FEMALE BULLIES AND FEMI-NAZIS
FEMALE CARNALITY
FEMALE DUMB DOWN
FEMALE POWER DRIVE
FEMINISM AND RUIN 1 & 2
FIX FOR MISFITS
FOOLS & TRAMPS
FREEDOM SPEAKING
FRENEMY ENABLER
FRENEMY LIAR
FRENEMY THIEF
FRENEMY TRAITOR
TRENEMY TYRANT
GENIUS IS HELD DOWN
GLOBALISLAM
GOD USES THE FLAWED
HAZE OF THE LATTER DAYS

THE HERD IN WORDS
HIX POLITIX
HOW THEY RUINED US
JUST SKIP DINNER
LE FEMME AND THE COMMUNIST SPIRIT
LIBERAL CHAOS & ROT
LIBERAL DOUBLETHINK
LIBERAL GALL 1 & 2
LIBERAL SHOVE-DOWNS
LOCK YOUR GATE
LOSERS and Femme Fatales
MANUAL FOR SUPERIOR MEN
MODERN ART FROM HELL
MOSTLY FAKE
NOTES TO CHAMPS 1 & 2
OVERCOME FRENEMIES
PC MAKES US CRAZY
PEOPLE ARE CRUEL
PEOPLE PROBLEMS 1 & 2
PERSECUTED GENIUIS
POLI-PSYCH MYSTERIES
PRETENTIOUS SLOBS
QUEEN BEE
RED NEW DEAL
RETURNING TO FIRST NATURE
SEASON OF TREASON
SEPARATE MEANS HOLY
SOCIAL HYPNOTISM
SOLITUDE SOLUTION
SUPERCILIOUS
THE SCHOOLS SCREWED EM UP
TOAD TO PRINCE
TRIALS CYCLES
TRUMP VS. GROUP
TRUST IN TRASH
THE TRUTH ABOUT PEOPLE
UNDERHEANDEDLY CLEVER
WALK TALL WITHIN WALLS
WE'RE NOT ALL ONE
WINNERS SKIP DINNER
WORK OR SMERK

AUTHOR BIO
Karen Kellock Ph.D.

Ph.D Political Psychology, UCI 1976
Post-Doctoral: UCI Medical School
Department of Psychiatry
Grants NIMH, NIAAA

Ph.D. dissertation "A Systems-Theoretic View of Pathologic Interaction" made an early mark as the "Wife of the Alcoholic Syndrome". Postdoctoral research at UCI Medical, Dept. of Psychiatry on the systems surrounding pathology on NIMH and NIAAA federal grants: *The Contagion of Madness: The Psychology of Neurotic Interaction and Pathological Systems*. Therapy tool Therapeutic Playwriting introduced the play *Mary and Murv: Gruesome Twosomes in the Alcoholic Marriage*. She taught Abnormal Psychology and Pathological Systems Theory at UC and CSU campuses and developed "the Debris Theory of Disease" in five books and website: (www.karenkellock.org): *Champion Guides, Daily Fastarian, Just Skip Dinner, Arts of Paleo Fasting, Ageless Cornucopia. Manual for Superior Men is a* pick-it-up-anywhere book that you can't put down (20,000 Kellockialisms) and ever on your desktop it should be found (or this Ebook for superior wordsearch of new jargon).

www.ingramcontent.com/pod-product-compliance
Lightning Source LLC
Chambersburg PA
CBHW061751250726
48657CB00001B/67